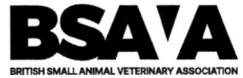

W0071721

BSAVA Guide to
Nutrition
in Small Animal Practice

Author:

Georgia Woods-Lee
BSc(Hons) RVN CertCFVHNut VTS(Nutrition)
Institute of Life Course & Medical Sciences and School of Veterinary Science,
University of Liverpool, Leahurst Campus, Chester High Road, Neston CH64 7TE

Editors:

Marge Chandler
DVM MS MANZCVS DipACVIM (Internal Medicine and Nutrition) MRCVS
Glasgow, Scotland

Alexander J. German
BVSc PhD CertSAM DipECVIM-CA SFHEA FRCVS
Institute of Life Course & Medical Sciences and School of Veterinary Science,
University of Liverpool, Leahurst Campus, Chester High Road, Neston CH64 7TE

Published by:

British Small Animal Veterinary Association
Woodrow House, 1 Telford Way,
Waterwells Business Park, Quedgeley,
Gloucester GL2 2AB

A Company Limited by Guarantee in England
Registered Company No. 2837793
Registered as a Charity

MIX
Paper | Supporting
responsible forestry
FSC® C016278

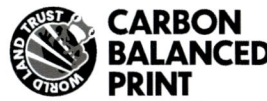

CARBON
BALANCED
PRINT
www.carbonbalancedprint.com
CBP2278

A catalogue record for this book is available from the British Library.

ISBN: Print: 978-1-913859-39-8 • Online: 978-1-913859-58-9
ePDF: 978-1-913859-37-4 • EPUB: 978-1-913859-38-1

Printed in the UK by Halstan & Co Ltd., Amersham HP6 6HJ

Titles in the BSAVA Manuals series:

Manual of Avian Practice: A Foundation Manual
Manual of Backyard Poultry Medicine and Surgery
Manual of Canine & Feline Abdominal Imaging
Manual of Canine & Feline Abdominal Surgery
Manual of Canine & Feline Advanced Veterinary Nursing
Manual of Canine & Feline Anaesthesia and Analgesia
Manual of Canine & Feline Behavioural Medicine
Manual of Canine & Feline Cardiorespiratory Medicine
Manual of Canine & Feline Clinical Pathology
Manual of Canine & Feline Dentistry and Oral Surgery
Manual of Canine & Feline Dermatology
Manual of Canine & Feline Emergency and Critical Care
Manual of Canine & Feline Endocrinology
Manual of Canine & Feline Endoscopy and Endosurgery
Manual of Canine & Feline Fracture Repair and Management
Manual of Canine & Feline Gastroenterology
Manual of Canine & Feline Haematology and Transfusion Medicine
Manual of Canine & Feline Head, Neck and Thoracic Surgery
Manual of Canine & Feline Musculoskeletal Disorders
Manual of Canine & Feline Musculoskeletal Imaging
Manual of Canine & Feline Nephrology and Urology
Manual of Canine & Feline Neurology
Manual of Canine & Feline Oncology
Manual of Canine & Feline Ophthalmology
Manual of Canine & Feline Radiography and Radiology: A Foundation Manual
Manual of Canine & Feline Rehabilitation, Supportive and Palliative Care
Manual of Canine & Feline Reproduction and Neonatology
Manual of Canine & Feline Shelter Medicine
Manual of Canine & Feline Surgical Principles: A Foundation Manual
Manual of Canine & Feline Thoracic Imaging
Manual of Canine & Feline Ultrasonography
Manual of Canine & Feline Wound Management and Reconstruction
Manual of Canine Practice: A Foundation Manual
Manual of Exotic Pet and Wildlife Nursing
Manual of Exotic Pets: A Foundation Manual
Manual of Feline Practice: A Foundation Manual
Manual of Practical Animal Care
Manual of Practical Veterinary Nursing
Manual of Practical Veterinary Welfare
Manual of Psittacine Birds
Manual of Rabbit Medicine
Manual of Rabbit Surgery, Dentistry and Imaging
Manual of Raptors, Pigeons and Passerine Birds
Manual of Reptiles
Manual of Rodents and Ferrets
Manual of Small Animal Practice Management and Development
Manual of Wildlife Casualties

**For further information on these and all BSAVA publications,
please visit our website: www.bsava.com**

Contents

Foreword

This new print edition of the *BSAVA Guide to Nutrition in Small Animal Practice* will be a valuable addition to your practice library. Expanding on the online version to give more advice on nutrition for specific diseases and life stages, it is very easy to read and crammed full of interesting and useful information.

The guide is divided into five clear sections and is augmented by online resources such as printable owner factsheets and helpful videos. The content is both practical and pragmatic, giving clear advice to vets and nurses on how best to advise owners on the different types of food available and how to calculate the amounts of food to be given.

Nutrition is regarded as the fifth vital assessment, alongside temperature, pulse, respiration and pain. It is vital then that vets and nurses know the correct questions to ask owners regarding the nutrition of their pet, as well as the correct answers to give regarding the same. Owners will frequently come to us for advice on the amount of food to give, or else will tell us about a new diet that they are using. This guide lays out how we could improve these conversations, as well as the advice we give, and thus strengthen our bonds with clients.

There are six chapters dealing with diet type – ranging from commercially manufactured diets to alternative protein-based diets. Each of these chapters includes advantages and disadvantages of the diet, safety measures and considerations such as cost and sustainability, enabling the client to make a truly informed decision about what to feed their pet.

What really stands out to me is the level of detail included in the guide: there is ample explanation of the underlying principles of nutrition, as well as formulae for specific nutritional plans. Where there may be confusion, or potential errors in calculating nutritional requirements, there are practical hints and tips for avoiding those pitfalls. Clearly, the guide has been put together by a panel who are very competent in their field and wish for the reader to become confident and competent as well.

Julian Hoad
BSc(Hons) BVetMed HonMBVNA MRCVS
BSAVA President 2024–5)

Preface

The topic of providing nutrition for cats and dogs is vast, with an ever changing and evolving landscape. Peppered with differences of opinion, and conflicting advice and evidence, it can be difficult for veterinary professionals to discuss and implement the ideal nutritional recommendation.

The *BSAVA Guide to Nutrition in Small Animal Practice* firstly aims to bring clarity to the subject so that veterinary professionals can have balanced, evidenced-based discussions with pet owners. As these discussions are frequently lengthy, additional resources have been included to enhance the degree of pet owner understanding with printable client handouts to reiterate the information given during consultations. In a world of high social media use where misinformation seems to live and breed, the guide aims to bring together all current evidence and best practice in an easy to read and practical manner. This makes it not only a trusted resource to share with pet owners, but a valuable addition to any practice library.

The guide secondly aims to provide answers for veterinary professionals looking to provide an excellent nutritional recommendation to all patients under their care. It covers all life stages and key diseases where nutrition has an influential or pivotal role. Further, each chapter examines the current evidence, providing important references and highlights where additional work is needed, whilst myth busting some commonly held ideas and beliefs.

I would like to give my heartfelt thanks to both of the editors, Marge Chandler and Alexander German, without whom this book would not have been possible. Your knowledge on nutrition topics and your passion for the subject remains a huge inspiration to me, and I count myself very fortunate to have received your guidance and mentorship. Finally, I would also like to thank the publishing team at BSAVA, your support and patience has been invaluable.

Georgia Woods-Lee
BSc(Hons) RVN CertCFVHNut VTS(Nutrition)

July 2025

The importance of nutrition   1

Nutrition is the cornerstone of good health and wellbeing for pets. Through decades of innovation, research and development, there are now many excellent diets to feed pets that are safe and which will deliver everything a pet needs in optimal quantities. For healthy pets, the aim of these diets is to maintain good health and quality of life for as long as possible. When nutritional requirements change in times of illness or disease, the aim is to support the pet on their return to good health, or aid in the management of their disease. In recent years, the development of disease-specific dietetic food has increased. These not only deliver essential nutritional requirements but also have nutritional adaptations to help reduce signs or the impact of diseases and promote recovery. Nutritional management of disease complements other medical management (e.g. pharmaceuticals). To deliver optimal nutrition for each disease state, an understanding of disease aetiology and pathology is required.

To provide an appropriate recommendation, all nutritional requirements should be considered. Whatever the type of food the owner chooses to feed, it should meet recommendations by the European Pet Food Industry Federation (FEDIAF, 2024) and the Association of American Feed Control Officials (AAFCO, 2018) to accommodate differences in digestibility and nutrient interactions (see below) and fulfil all nutritional aims (Figure 1.1).

Nutritional aims	Comments
Complete and balanced nutrition	The diet should provide every nutrient that the pet needs in the correct quantities and not in excessive amounts
Digestible	The nutrients must be bioavailable to the pet consuming the food
Palatable	The food must be appealing to the pet so that they will consume it. Factors affecting palatability include: ■ Fats ■ Moisture ■ Protein ■ Aroma ■ Texture
Not fed in excess	Excessive amounts of energy from any food will lead to obesity (see Chapter 15). Controlling the amount of food is strongly advised to maintain an ideal body condition score

Figure 1.1: Nutritional aims that should be met by all types of diet. (continues) ▶

Nutritional aims	Comments
Safe	The food must be safe to feed, being free from anything that may cause harm to the pet, pet owner or other individuals who have contact with the pet (e.g. toxic compounds or organisms that cause disease)
Achievable	The recommendation must be manageable for the pet owner and should take into consideration: ■ Financial budget ■ Available time ■ Motivation level ■ Accessibility to the food (e.g. being able to collect it in person or order it online for delivery. Not all pet owners will have suitable transport or have the equipment and capabilities to order food digitally)
Sustainability	The sustainability of food sources is of increasing concern for both humans and pets because if current consumption continues, there will be a food shortage within the next 50 years (see Chapters 7 and 8)

Figure 1.1: (continued) Nutritional aims that should be met by all types of diet.

Feeding trials (Beaton, 2022) assess how animals respond to a type of food over a period of time and should take into account AAFCO guidelines including:

- Number of animals – at least eight healthy animals at least 1 year of age
- Test duration – 6 months
- Veterinary examination – a complete examination should to be conducted at beginning and end of the trial
- Blood test – should be undertaken at the beginning and end of the trial for specific parameters
- Weight monitoring – animals should be weighed weekly
  - Animals cannot lose more than 15% of their bodyweight
  - Average weight loss of the group cannot be more than 10%.
- Food consumption – animals may only consume the food being tested.

Digestibility testing (Bos *et al.*, 2023) uses standardized conditions to assess how well a dog food is digested. Current protocols when using an indigestible marker include:

- Six healthy fully grown dogs over 1 year of age
- A study period of between 7 days (FEDIAF) and 10 days (AAFCO) including an adaptation period and a faecal collection period (AAFCO requires 5 days, whereas FEDIAF only recommend 3 days based on a single study; Nott *et al.*, 1994).

Barriers to optimal nutrition provision

There are several reasons that make optimal nutrition difficult to achieve, including:

- Choice
  - A wide range of diet types are available making it confusing for pet owners to decide.

- Differing levels of knowledge and education
- Differing sources of information
  - Owners may seek advice from veterinary professionals, breeders, the internet, books, newspapers and magazines, media or friends or use previous experience to inform their decision.
- Minimal evidence for many of the types of food available
- Differences in opinion about what constitutes an optimal diet for dogs and cats
- Conflicting advice amongst sources of information, resulting in confusion.

Nutritional safety

Whether commercially produced pet food, home-prepared cooked food or raw food is provided, it is recommended that recipes are created or approved by an appropriately qualified individual.

Appropriate qualifications

These include:

- PhD in animal nutrition
- Diploma from the American College of Veterinary Internal Medicine (ACVIM – Nutrition)
- Diploma from the European College of Veterinary Comparative Nutrition (ECVCN).

Many of the larger pet food manufacturers employ such qualified individuals full time. Some formulations are fixed formula recipes, whereby manufacturers can guarantee product consistency meaning that there is little variation amongst batches. Others use variable formula (or open formula) diets, which are less expensive; however, the ingredients of such diets may change from batch to batch, reflecting variations in the cost and availability of ingredients to the producer. Although uncommon, variations in ingredients can have negative effects on pets who are less tolerant of dietary changes, potentially resulting in gastrointestinal disturbances or other adverse reactions to food.

Information on the type of formulation used can be obtained from the manufacturer and some details may be printed on the pet food label. Some label information must be displayed for legal reasons, whereas other information is for marketing purposes (Figure 1.2).

Product safety

Hygiene

Basic hygiene is essential for the safe feeding of any diet to prevent contamination with pathogens.

- Containers and packaging should be inspected for any damage or contamination that may affect the food. Any product with damaged packaging should not be purchased and should be discarded.
- Effective hand hygiene is important before and after food preparation.
- Preparation areas and surfaces should be cleaned before and after food is prepared.
- Clean food bowls should be used for each meal.
- Bowls and utensils should be washed after feeding.
- Bowls or plates for pet use should be kept separate from the ones used by the owners.

Interpreting Food Labels, EU

Net weight must be reported

The pet food label must:
- Specify target species and lifestage
- Specify if the food is "complete" (provides all necessary nutrients and energy for the species and lifestage, and can be used as sole source of nutrition) or "complementary" (does not provide all nutrients and mainly refers to treats)

Feeding instructions can be more or less detailed. Many labels state that these are only recommendations and might vary depending on age, breed, activity and health

Label should include storage instructions (canned food might also include storage instructions after opening)

Dry pet food must recommend that the pet must have fresh water available at all times

[Product name]   400 g

Complete pet food
for adult cats

Composition: Meat and animal derivatives (4% chicken), vegetable protein extract, derivatives of vegetable origin, cereals, minerals, various sugars

weight (kg)	serving / day (g)
2	35
3	50
4	62
5	74

Additives (per kg):
Nutritional additives:
Vitamin D3 xx UI, E1
(Iron) xx mg [...].
Preservatives:
antioxidants

Store in a cool dry place

Analytical constituents: Crude protein XX %, Crude oils and fats XX %, Crude ash XX %, Crude fibres XX %, Moisture XX%

ABC (company responsible of labelling/packaging), address/phone #

BATCH 1234567890
plant ABCD
Best before date MM/YYYY

Ingredients (raw materials) are listed under "composition"

-In descending order of weight (fresh matter)
-The names can be specific or can also be named by their legal category (see example)

Label must include those nutritional additives (vitamins and minerals) with legal inclusion maximums. The amounts are those added (therefore, the overall amount of nutrient might be different depending on raw material provision and effect of processing. Other additives (like preservatives, dyes, or flavouring agents) do not have to be reported by their specific name, but the company responsible for labelling should provide this information if contacted.

Name, address and contact information of the company responsible for labelling must be included. Label does not have to include country of production. If it applies, companies can use "made in the EU"

Label should include traceability information such as batch number and plant approval number. Best before date must be included in month and year (plus day if short shelf life)

Analytical constituents are declared as percentages (grams per 100 g of pet food) in fresh matter. The ones that are mandatory are crude protein, crude oils and fats, crude ash, and crude fibres. Moisture is only mandatory if >14% . The energy density (kilocalories per kg, cup or can) is not mandatory and is often absent form labels.

Figure 1.2: WSAVA guidance for interpreting pet food labels.
(Reproduced with permission from the World Small Animal Veterinary Association)

Since some diet types pose a greater risk than others (e.g. those with uncooked ingredients), appropriate advice on feeding safety must be given when such diets are identified as being fed.

Communication with pet owners

Most owners want to do what is best for their pet. With the evidence available, veterinary professionals must, without prejudice, give the best advice possible to ensure that the pet receives a complete and balanced diet. Veterinary professionals should separate what has been proven from advice based on clinical experience and reasoning. When talking to owners about different available diets, it is important to understand their motivations, correct any misperceptions and provide them with appropriate guidance so that they can feed their pet optimally and safely. Pet owners should be discouraged from searching the internet for treatments or supplements which have no scientific evidence of effectiveness. Should a change in diet be recommended, pet owners should receive tailored guidance on how to transition from one diet to another successfully, without causing adverse effects (see Chapter 2). It is vital that the transition is not rushed; in most cases there is no time pressure to make the diet transition.

Conclusion

There is now a wide array of diets available for dogs and cats, including those with various illnesses, meaning that a suitable diet can be chosen for most pets, whether to sustain good health or to assist with recovery from injury or therapy for disease. Provided a diet satisfies all the necessary criteria, it can be recommended to pet owners, ideally working with the owner and acknowledging their preferences (see Chapter 2).

References and further reading

AAFCO (2018) *Official publication*. [Available from: https://www.aafco.org/resources/official-publication/]

Beaton L (2022) The expectations and limitations of feeding trials. *PetFood Industry*. [Available from: https://www.petfoodindustry.com/pet-food-market/article/15468983/the-expectations-and-limitations-of-feeding-trials#:~:text=Learn%20about%20the%20expectations%20and,information%20possible%20from%20their%20research.&text=The%20Association%20of%20American%20Feed,for%20the%20six%2Dmonth%20duration.]

Bos E, Hendriks W, Beerda B and Bosch G (2023) Determining the protocol requirements of in-home dog food digestibility testing. *British Journal of Nutrition* **130(1)**, 164–173

Commission Regulation (EU) 2020/354 (2020) *Establishing a list of intended uses of feed intended for particular nutritional purposes and repealing Directive 2008/38/EC*. [Available from: https://eur-lex.europa.eu/legal-content/EN/TXT/?uri=CELEX:32020R0354]

FEDIAF (2024) *Nutritional guidelines for complete and complementary pet food for cats and dogs*. [Available from: https://europeanpetfood.org/wp-content/uploads/2024/09/FEDIAF-Nutritional-Guidelines_2024.pdf]

Food Standards Agency (2017) *Business Guidance – Pet Food*. [Available from: www.food.gov.uk/business-guidance/pet-food]

Food Standards Agency (2018) *Avondale Pet Foods Ltd recalls Just Natural Chicken and Tripe because Salmonella has been found in the produce*. [Available from: www.food.gov.uk/news-alerts/alert/fsa-prin-71-2018]

Food Standards Agency (2019a) *Raw Treat Pet Food Ltd recalls frozen raw beef, chicken, lamb, and chicken and tripe pet food due to the presence of Listeria monocytogenes*.

[Available from: www.food.gov.uk/news-alerts/alert/fsa-prin-36-2019]

Food Standards Agency (2019b) *Raw Treat Pet Food Ltd recalls varieties of frozen raw pet food due to the presence of Salmonella.* [Available from: www.food.gov.uk/news-alerts/alert/fsa-prin-38-]

Hill's Pet Nutrition (2019) *Important voluntary product recall information.* [Available from: www.hillspet.co.uk/productlist]

O'Halloran C, Ioannidi O, Reed N *et al.* (2019) Tuberculosis due to *Mycobacterium bovis* in pet cats associated with feeding a commercial raw food diet. *Journal of Feline Medicine and Surgery* **21(8)**, 667–681

People's Dispensary for Sick Animals (2019) *PDSA Animal Wellbeing Report (PAW) Report.* [Available from: www.pdsa.org.uk/media/7420/2019-paw-report_ downloadable.pdf]

Pet Food Manufacturers' Association (2015) *Pets at Home recall.* [Available from: www.pfma.org.uk/news/pets-at-home-recall]

US Food and Drug Administration (2007) *Melamine Pet Food Recall.* [Available from: www.fda.gov/animal-veterinary/recalls-withdrawals/melamine-pet-food-recall-frequently-asked-questions]

Woods-Lee G (2025) *BSAVA Guide to Nutrition in Small Animal Practice – owner factsheets,* ed. AJ German and M Chandler. [Available from: www.bsavalibrary.com/nutritionguide]

Useful websites

American College of Veterinary Internal Medicine (ACVIM)

https://www.acvim.org/about-acvim/acvn-redirect

European College of Veterinary and Comparative Nutrition (ECVCN)

https://www.ecvcn.org/

European Pet Food Industry Federation (FEDIAF)

https://europeanpetfood.org/

Nutritional assessment

2

Providing a suitable diet is one of the five welfare needs for which a pet owner is responsible (Animal Welfare Act, 2006). Provision of food that the pet enjoys eating will be of vital importance because, to owners, this is an important sign of health and wellbeing. Given that there are many different food types, brands and specific diets available, there can be great variety amongst pets in what is actually consumed.

Initial nutritional assessment

Alongside evaluation of temperature, pulse, respiration and pain, nutrition is now considered to be the fifth vital assessment (Pet Nutrition Alliance, 2014). A nutritional assessment assesses all aspects of feeding, facilitating evaluation of both the diet and feeding management. It is critical that veterinary professionals understand what foods are being fed to ensure that the diet fulfils all nutritional aims, and to provide suitable advice if it does not (see Chapter 1). Decisions owners make about what to feed their pet will usually have been made with the best intentions; albeit not always based on reliable information. In one study, 90% of pet owners stated that they would have welcomed a nutritional assessment by the healthcare team, but only 15% received one (Pet Nutrition Alliance, 2014).

A thorough nutritional assessment can take time. Information needs to be gathered efficiently; asking owners to complete a pre-appointment questionnaire can be useful (Figure 2.1). Such assessment forms can be handed to the owner in the waiting room or provided ahead of the appointment. Whatever format is selected, the ease of use and access to the necessary technology, if needed, should be considered. The information gathered via the questionnaire can then be reviewed and discussed with the owner during their appointment.

Key information to obtain during an initial nutritional assessment includes:

- Pet and owner identity
- Species and breed
- Age (in months and years)
- Sex
- Neutered status
- Pattern and amount of activity
- Weight and body condition
  - Oral health/teeth
  - Skin and coat condition
- Current food
  - Brand
  - Type (e.g. wet food, home-prepared or proprietary)
  - Quantity of food and how this is measured (e.g. scales, cup, handful)

BSAVA Client Handouts: Nutrition Guide Series

Nutritional Assessment Form

Owner details

Name	
Address	
Contact number	
Email address	

A downloadable form is available for this guide from the BSAVA library

Pet details

Pet's name	
Species	
Breed	
Age	
Sex	
Neutered (Y/N)	
Current weight Kg	Kg
Current body condition score (using a 9-point scales)	/9
Ideal bodyweight	Kg
Muscle condition score (Tick as appropriate)	Normal
	Mild wasting
	Moderate wasting
	Severe wasting
Activity level (Tick as appropriate)	High
	Moderate
	Low
Appetite (Tick as appropriate)	Normal
	Excessive
	Low

Food, treats, supplements

Current foods: List all brands/ prepared at home	Form: e.g Wet, dry, moist, fresh, frozen	Quantity per day	Current treats and chews: List all brands	Quantity per day

How is food measured out?	Handfuls
	Cup/scoop
	Weighing scales
Current supplements used	
Cats only	Catches and consumes prey? (Y/N)
Drinks consumed	

Additional notes:

Initials of person completing the form

Internal use only: Date form completed

©BSAVA 2025

BSAVA Guide to Nutrition in Small Animal Practice

Figure 2.1: An example of a nutritional assessment form.

- Number of meals per day
- How long the food has been fed
  - Previous food fed
- Purchased treats or chews
- Human foods used as treats
- Nutritional supplements
- Drinks (e.g. water, milk, soup)
- Feeding management (e.g. timing, competition, meal frequency)
- Housing
- Appetite
- Body condition score
- Muscle condition score.

Hospitalized patients
A nutritional assessment is vital for gathering information about hospitalized patients and will help facilitate the development of an individualized nutrition plan (see below).

Extended nutritional evaluation

In some cases, an extended evaluation may be required (Figure 2.2). Possible reasons for such an evaluation include:

- Life stages (e.g. gestation, lactation, growth, senior)
- Activity levels (very low or high)
- Abnormal body condition score (i.e. below ideal weight (<4 dogs) or above ideal weight (>5 for dogs and either >5 or >6 for some cats on a 9-point scale); see Chapter 15)
- Poor muscle condition score (see Chapter 11)
- Unexplained weight changes
- Presence of systemic disease
- Poor coat and skin quality
- Dental abnormalities or disease
- Receiving medication (prescribed or otherwise)
- Receiving nutritional supplements (veterinary recommended or otherwise)
- Unconventional diet type
- Poorly balanced and incomplete diets delivering >10% of calories
- Disrupted gastrointestinal function
- Treats that exceed 10% of dietary intake
- Altered gastrointestinal function (e.g. vomiting, diarrhoea, constipation).

Further points to consider during an extended nutritional assessment include:

- Interactions with other household pets or family members
- Any behavioural concerns
- Where the pet spends most of its time (e.g. indoors or outdoors)
- Information on any risk factors that have been identified during the initial nutritional assessment.

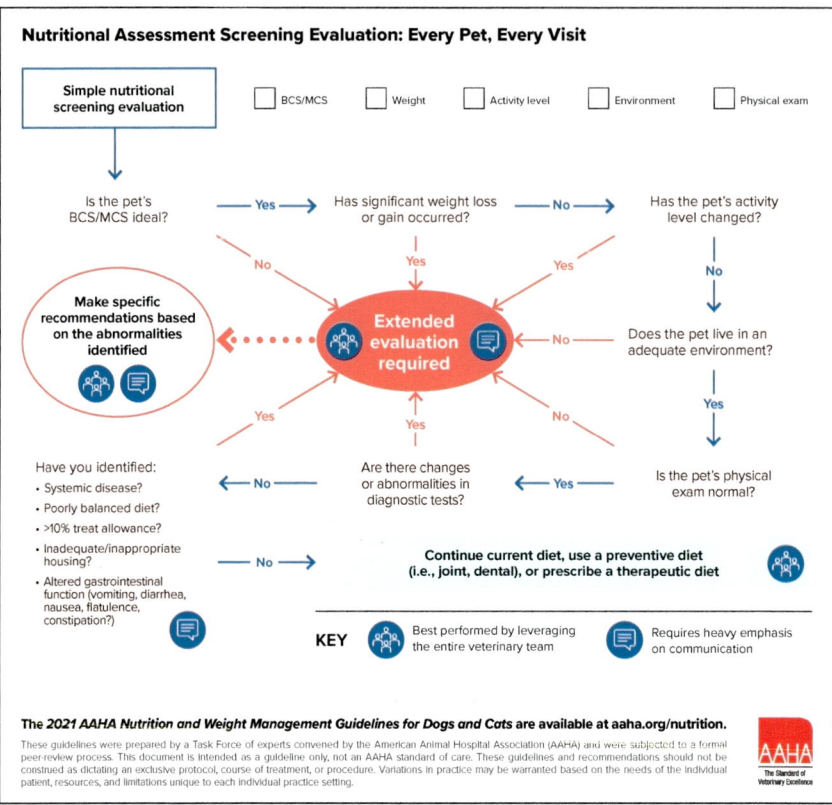

Figure 2.2: Factors that should be considered when determining whether an extended nutritional evaluation is required.
(Reproduced with permission from the American Animal Hospital Association)

Formulating a plan

The aim of formulating a plan and providing a nutritional recommendation is to ensure optimal nutrition for each individual pet. The diet selected will depend on the information obtained during the initial nutritional assessment in conjunction with information from the extended evaluation, if performed. Even if the current main diet is adequate, it may still be necessary to advise small alterations, especially with regards to additional foods (e.g. treats) or supplements the pet may be receiving. Where appropriate, the owner should be commended for good diet choice and feeding management. Once a suitable food has been identified, the next step is to calculate the expected daily energy intake for the animal and the amount of food needed to provide this. As many possible calculations can be used to estimate energy requirements, it is preferable to agree a single method for all practice staff to use. It should be noted that as these calculations are estimates, the required calories for an individual pet can vary by as much as 50 percent. Adjustments should be made as necessary to maintain a good body condition score.

Calculations

There are two main calculations for daily energy requirements for cats and dogs. The maintenance energy requirement (MER) is used to estimate the normal daily calorie requirement for pets at home. The resting energy requirement (RER) is used to estimate the daily calorie requirement for hospitalized patients where their energy requirement is significantly reduced due to inactivity. Another useful calculation for hospitalized patients is the daily energy requirement (DER), which can be used for staged reintroduction to food (e.g. assisted feeding) following a prolonged period of anorexia (see Chapter 13).

Maintenance energy requirement

- Dogs: 95 x bodyweight $^{0.75}$ = kcal/day
  (consider increasing this amount by 10–30% if the dog is known to be physically active (e.g. a working or agility dog))
- Cats (lean): 100 x bodyweight $^{0.67}$ = kcal/day
- Cats (obese or prone to obesity): 130 x bodyweight $^{0.4}$ = kcal/day
  (Note: this calculation is used to determine maintenance energy requirements in cats with obesity and not the amount required to induce controlled weight reduction; for more information on controlled weight reduction, see Chapter 15)

Examples:
- **20 kg dog**
  - $95 \times 20^{0.75}$ = 899 kcal/day
- **3.5 kg cat (lean)**
  - $100 \times 3.5^{0.67}$ = 232 kcal/day
- **5 kg cat (obese)**
  - $130 \times 5^{0.4}$ = 248 kcal/day

Note: To perform these calculations, a scientific calculator should be used. For $^{0.67}$ the x^y symbol should be used (e.g. type 100×3.5 x^y 0.67 = to get the answer). Use rounded numbers for ease of feeding

Resting energy requirement

- For patients weighing 2–30 kg: (bodyweight x 30) + 70 = kcal/day
- For all patients (including those weighing <2 kg or >30 kg): 70 x bodyweight $^{0.75}$ = kcal/day

Examples:
- **15 kg dog**
  - (15×30) + 70 = 450 + 70 = 520 kcal/day
- **1.5 kg cat**
  - $70 \times 1.5^{0.75}$ = 95 kcal/day
- **32 kg dog**
  - $70 \times 32^{0.75}$ = 942 kcal/day

Note: To perform these calculations, a scientific calculator should be used. For $^{0.75}$ the x^y symbol should be used (e.g. type 70×32 x^y 0.75 = to get the answer).

Pet food labels explained

Owners will often seek guidance about whether a food they have sourced is suitable for their pet, but this can be a difficult question to answer. Pet food labels contain legal, regulated information, product marketing text and images (see Chapter 1). Labels usually include feeding guidelines based on the weight of the pet, or age if feeding kitten or puppy food. The calorie content is rarely printed on the labels because there is no legal requirement to do so in the United Kingdom (UK). The analytical constituents information can be used to estimate how much food to feed per day. This means a daily feeding allocation can be swiftly estimated for any diet.

Calculating calorie content from food labels

To calculate the calorie content of any commercially manufactured food, the percentage of the analytical constituents including protein, fat, ash, fibre, moisture in the food (unless otherwise stated, the moisture content of dry food is estimated to be approximately 10%) and carbohydrate is needed. However, the percentage content of carbohydrate is not usually printed on the packaging, so this will need to be calculated (see below). The estimated calorie content of the food can then be calculated based on the metabolizable energy (ME) of protein, fat and carbohydrate (see below).

To calculate carbohydrate content:
- 100% - (% protein + % fat + % ash + % fibre + % moisture) = % carbohydrate content

Examples:
- Dry food:
  - $100 - (31 + 20 + 9.3 + 1.8 + 10) = 100 - 72.1 = 27.9\%$ carbohydrate
- Wet food:
  - $100 - (7.8 + 5.0 + 1.5 + 83.5) = 100 - 97.8 = 2.2\%$ carbohydrate

To calculate calorie content using the metabolizable energy (UK Pet Food, 2015):
- % protein x 3.5 = kcal/100 g
- % fat x 8.5 = kcal/100 g
- % carbohydrate x 3.5 = kcal/100 g
- Add all three together = total calories in food/100 g

Examples:
- Dry food:
  - Protein: $31 \times 3.5 = 108.5$ kcal/100 g
  - Fat: $20 \times 8.5 = 170$ kcal/100 g
  - Carbohydrate: $27.9 \times 3.5 = 97.65$ kcal/100 g
  - Total calories: $108.5 + 170 + 97.65 = 376.15$ kcal/100 g
- Wet food:
  - Protein: $7.8 \times 3.5 = 98$ kcal/100 g
  - Fat: $5.0 \times 8.5 = 42.5$ kcal/100 g
  - Carbohydrate: $2.2 \times 3.5 = 7.7$ kcal/100 g
  - Total calories: $98 + 42.5 + 7.7 = 148.2$ kcal/100g

Note: whilst this is a relatively straightforward method, it is not perfect. More accurate, albeit more complex, calculations have also been devised (e.g. those recommended by the National Research Council, 2006)

Meal split

The number of meals pets are fed per day can vary greatly; some are offered food just once daily whilst others are fed more frequently and/or fed *ad libitum* (freely). When making a recommendation, it is useful to know how many meals the owner wishes to feed. If a mixed diet of dry and wet food is fed, the amount of each needs to be calculated. The number of units of wet food fed per day (e.g. pouches, tins) should first be determined, with the remaining calories used for the dry food component.

Examples:
- **20 kg dog fed 1 tin of wet food per day with dry food**
  - RER = 662 kcal/day
  - 1 tin of wet food = 336 kcal
    662 – 336 = 326 kcal remaining
  - 1 g of dry food = 3.76 kcal
    326 / 3.76 = 87 g of dry food per day
- **3.5 kg cat fed 2 pouches per day with dry food**
  - RER = 179 kcal/day
  - 1 pouch = 56 kcal x 2 = 112 kcal
    179 – 112 = 67 kcal remaining
  - 1 g of dry food = 3.5 kcal
    67 / 3.5 = 19 g of dry food per day

Calculating cost to feed per day

Some owners might be concerned about the cost of pet food, and this can be the reason for one diet being selected over another. This is of greater concern if a dietetic food has been advised (e.g. weight loss diet, renal diet).

Calculating cost of food per day:
- Amount in bag (g) / ration per day (g) = number of days bag will last
- Price of food (£) / days bag will last = cost per day (£)

Example:
- 1500 g / 45 g per day = 33 days
- £14 / 33 = £0.42 per day

Calculating the cost of food per meal:
- Cost per day (£) / number of meals = cost per meal (£)

Example:
- £0.42 / 2 = £0.21 per meal

Transitioning to a new food

It is important to give owners advice on how to introduce a new food to their pet. A gradual transition should always be recommended as this will help prevent gastric disturbances and ensure acceptance of the new food. The new food should be introduced slowly over a period of time by replacing amounts of the old food with the new. There is no correct duration for such transition, although some suggestions are given in Figure 2.3.

Category	Transition time	Guidance
Readily eat anything offered	3 days	A pet who has a healthy appetite, readily accepts new foods or is very food focused and is described as 'will eat anything', may be transitioned to a new food over a few days to prevent digestive disturbance
Good eaters	4–7 days	Pets who are usually good eaters but may need a slightly slower approach to allow for better acceptance of new foods should be transitioned over a slightly longer time to promote acceptance and prevent digestive disturbance
Picky eaters	10–14 days	A slower transition would be best for those pets that are wary about new foods or who may have refused new foods in the past. The extended transition promotes acceptance and prevents digestive disturbance. The transition must not be rushed in these cases
Fussy eaters	2–3 weeks or more	Pets that do not adapt well to changes to their food, or where a food transition has previously failed, should have a very slow transition with only minimal amounts of food changed at a time. This may also be needed if the new food is very different from the previously fed diet. If necessary, these pets should be introduced to only one kibble or teaspoonful of the new food per day. It may take up to 2 months in some cases to successfully complete a food transition (Ross *et al.*, 2006)

Figure 2.3: Guidance on transition times for new food introduction.

Communication with pet owners

To obtain the most information from discussions with pet owners, open (rather than closed) questions should be used. Owners are likely to describe only what the pet eats for their main meals, and may not volunteer information on other foods, treats or supplements unless specifically asked. Using a phrase such as 'starting first thing in the morning, tell me everything your pet eats before you go to bed' has been shown to elicit more useful and relevant information (Coe *et al.*, 2020).

It is important that the pet owner feels comfortable discussing the information and does not feel judged by the veterinary team with regards to the food or quantity of treats. Trust and rapport are essential parts of the veterinary professional–pet owner relationship. It should be remembered that whatever the owner is feeding it is likely to be based (rightly or wrongly) on what they believe to be best for their pet. Therefore, the owner should be first reassured that the more information they provide, the better the individualized nutritional recommendation will be.

Should the current diet be found to be unsuitable for the pet, owners can be informed of any risks and either how to make the food safer, or possible alternatives. In such situations, a range of alternatives should be suggested to enable the owner to make the ultimate decision.

Conclusion

A nutritional assessment should be undertaken for every pet during every consultation; it is a key tool in providing excellent veterinary healthcare and allows for individualized nutritional recommendations. Without a nutritional assessment, dietary deficiencies may not be identified and cases where a specific diet may be beneficial to the health of the pet may be missed. Establishing a relationship with the owners based on trust and support will mean that the best nutritional solution can be found for their pet.

References and further reading

Animal Welfare Act (2006) [Available from: https://www.legislation.gov.uk/ukpga/2006/45/contents]

Coe JB, O'Connor RE, MacMartin C, Verbrugghe A and Janke KA (2020) Effects of three diet history questions on the amount of information gained from a sample of pet owners in Ontario, Canada. *Journal of the American Veterinary Medical Association* **256**, 469–478

National Research Council (2006) Energy. In: *Nutrient Requirements of Dogs and Cats*. National Academic Press, Washington DC

Pet Nutrition Alliance (2014) *Tips for implementing nutrition as a vital assessment in your practice.* [Available from: https://wsava.org/wp-content/uploads/2020/01/Quick-Tips-on-Implementing-the-WSAVA-Nutrition-Guidelines.pdf]

Ross SJ, Osbourne CA, Kirk CA, Lowry SR, Koehler LA and Polzin DJ (2006) Clinical evaluation of dietary modification for treatment of spontaneous chronic kidney disease in cats. *Journal of the American Veterinary Medical Association* **229(6)**, 949–957

UK Pet Food (2015) *Calculating the energy content of prepared pet food and daily energy requirements of adult dogs and cats: factsheet.* [Available from: https://www.ukpetfood.org/spotlight-on-obesity/calculating-how-much-to-feed/calorie-calculating-fact-sheet.html]

Online extras

This chapter includes:

- **A nutritional assessment form that is available to download and print from the BSAVA Library. The form is marked in the text with a download symbol** ⬇

- **Videos of worked calculations**

Access via QR code or: bsavalibrary.com/nutrition_2

Commercially manufactured diets

3

Commercially manufactured diets, or proprietary diets, are pet foods produced on an industrial scale and widely distributed to stockists for convenient purchasing. They have been popular with pet owners for many years, with the first such diet for dogs being produced in the United Kingdom (UK) in 1860. Since this time, commercially manufactured diets have consistently risen in popularity. Now widely available, they offer many advantages to pet owners and veterinary professionals alike.

The diets, at every stage of production, are usually subjected to testing and analysis for nutritional adequacy, product consistency and pathogen elimination (although the extent and nature of this will depend on the diet and the manufacturing company). Many manufacturers also research dietary formulations, with purpose-formulated diets now available for specific life stages and medical conditions. This allows optimal nutrition (i.e. above the minimum nutritional requirements) to be delivered to pets.

Recipes for these diets are created by professional formulators trained in the commercial formulation of pet foods, in consultation with an appropriately qualified individual (see Chapter 1). In addition, many of the larger pet food manufacturers also undertake feeding trials and/or laboratory analyses to ensure that their diets deliver complete and balanced nutrition. Although conducting feeding trials (see Chapter 1) is very expensive, it is recognized as the gold standard method for determining nutrient availability. In the UK, the European Pet Food Industry Federation (FEDIAF, 2024) provides the nutrient guidelines that should be adhered to when formulating a diet. Nutrition should not be merely adequate but should be optimal for the pet consuming the food, meaning that commercially manufactured diets are frequently formulated to a specification superior to basic nutritional requirements.

It is possible for manufacturers to analyse the ingredients in the recipe used to create the diet in a laboratory setting to ensure that it contains the necessary nutrient concentrations – but there are some limitations to this method. The main drawback is that this method will not assess the level of bioavailability of the nutrient being consumed. In addition, manufacturers may only test the macronutrients within the diet, as testing for specific amino acids, vitamins and minerals can be expensive. Without knowing whether the intended recipient of the diet can digest and utilize the nutrients present, complete and balanced nutrition cannot be guaranteed to the same degree as for those diets tested by feeding trials. Smaller commercially manufactured diet producers will typically formulate their diets in this way. Many small pet food manufacturers use computer formulation software, without any laboratory analysis of the diet. It should be noted that in Europe, a claim that a diet is 'complete' can be based on a computer formulation alone, however, FEDIAF state in the guidelines that each product should be validated by chemical analysis of the finished product using an officially recognized method.

Types of commercially manufactured diet

Commercially manufactured diets are produced in three main forms: dry, wet and uncooked or raw meat-based diets (see Chapter 6). These forms differ depending on moisture content, intended preservation method and processing methods of the ingredients (Figure 3.1). Through scientific development, dietetic food is now available for a wide range of conditions, including renal disease, skin disease, diabetes mellitus, obesity and hyperthyroidism (Commission Regulation, 2020). For some conditions, the correct dietetic food can eliminate clinical signs of the disease.

Type of diet	Product details	Advantages

Dry foods (kibble)	■ Low moisture content (typically 3–11%)
	■ Generally higher starch content – necessary for the kibble to hold its shape
	■ Produced most commonly via an extrusion method:
	  • Uses pressure and temperature to rapidly cook the ingredients (20–60 seconds). It is widely used as it increases the digestibility and palatability of the food (Case *et al.*, 2000)
	  • Used to kill pathogenic bacteria
	■ Sold in bags of varying sizes (500 g to 15 kg)
		■ Cost-effective
		■ Proportionally less packaging needed so more environmentally friendly than wet products
		■ Can be produced rapidly in large volumes
		■ Distribution can be quick and effective, so foods are conveniently available to pet owners
		■ Suitable for all pets

Wet foods (chunks in gravy/jelly, loaf or pâté)	■ High moisture content (60–87%)
	■ Available in tins, trays and pouches
	■ Uses heat and pressure to preserve the ingredients, but each method depends on packaging type
		■ Increased palatability due to high moisture content. This can be advantageous for picky eaters; some pets may have a preference for other diet types
		■ A high moisture intake may be advantageous for:
		  • Senior cats
		  • Pets with specific diseases requiring increased water intake (e.g. renal disease (see Chapter 19) or lower urinary tract disease (see Chapter 20); Case, 2010)
		■ Often sold in single-serving packages, so food waste is low and fresh food can be given at each meal, promoting consistent palatability. However, this produces more packaging waste
		■ Cat owners prefer to provide mixed food to their pets, with 50% of cats now being fed some wet and some dry foods daily (PDSA, 2019)

Figure 3.1: The different types of available commercially manufactured diets and their advantages.(continues) ▶

Type of diet	Product details	Advantages

Uncooked foods	■ Variable moisture content depending on the specific diet
	   • Tend to have a higher moisture content (similar to wet foods)
	   • Dry foods with additional freeze-dried ingredients are also available. Ingredients are preserved by freezing or freeze-drying before thawing or rehydration prior to feeding
		■ Commercially manufactured uncooked products have some advantages compared with home-prepared raw diets (see Chapter 6) or home-prepared cooked diets (see Chapter 5), as they undergo freezing or freeze-drying, which decreases the *Campylobacter* colony count. However, this process will not completely eradicate Campylobacter or other pathogens, some of which are unaffected by freezing (van Bree *et al.*, 2018). It should be noted that the freezing of uncooked pet foods does not guarantee food safety
		■ High-pressure pasteurization is also used to reduce pathogenic risk; however, further research is required to determine its efficacy

Figure 3.1: (continued) The different types of available commercially manufactured diets and their advantages.

Advantages of feeding a commercially manufactured diet

- ■ Assured safety (see below)
  - There are regulations in place to govern production.
- ■ Low preparation time
  - There is no need for significant preparation of food and no cooking is required.
- ■ Balanced nutrition
  - Recipes are designed, overseen or approved by an appropriately qualified person (see Chapter 1). Commercial pet food manufacturers should be able to provide, on request, information on who has been involved in the process.
- ■ Good digestibility
  - All commercially manufactured diets should meet the minimum level of digestibility. This can be tested during feeding trials. Wet products are typically more digestible than dry foods.
- ■ Product consistency
  - Larger pet food manufacturers use fixed formula recipes, whereby they can guarantee product consistency meaning that there is little variation between batches. Other manufacturers use variable formula (or open formula) diets, which are less expensive; however, the ingredients of such diets may change from batch to batch, reflecting variations in the cost and availability of ingredients to the producer. Information on the type of formula used for a particular diet can be obtained from the manufacturer or pet food label (see Chapter 2).

- Good pet satisfaction
  - Satisfaction is guaranteed by many commercially manufactured diet producers through product consistency and high palatability.
- Convenience
  - Commercially manufactured diets can be purchased readily from various outlets (e.g. pet shops or supermarkets) and online. They are packaged to protect food from damage wherever possible and to ensure ease of storage.
- Variety
  - A wide variety of types and flavours are available. Pet owners are easily able to choose the flavour or type of food that their pet prefers.
- Cost effectiveness
  - Dry forms are the most cost-effective compared with other diet types (e.g. raw meat-based diets and home-prepared cooked diets). Wet diet types are often more expensive than dry.

Disadvantages of feeding a commercially manufactured diet

- High calorie content
  - Commercially manufactured dry diets usually have a greater energy content on a gram-for-gram basis than wet diets, which can increase the risk of overconsumption and lead to pet obesity if portions are not accurately weighed out (see Chapter 15).
    - An association between feeding dry food and overweight status has been identified in some (Öhlund *et al.*, 2018; Wall *et al.*, 2019) but not all (Robertson, 1999; Allan *et al.*, 2000; Russell *et al.*, 2000) of the epidemiological studies conducted in cats. Arguably, the overfeeding risk of leaving food out is more of a concern with dry food than wet food, partly because it is less liable to spoil (see below)
    - Dry food is approximately 4 times more energy dense that wet food, making it easier for the owner to overfeed, or the pet to over-consume. Unless the wet food contains a high fat content (e.g. 47%), cats typically consume 10–33% less energy when fed wet food (compared with dry food) *ad libiitum* (Jackson and Tovey, 1977; Tarttelin, 1987; Carciofi *et al.*, 2005).
- Prepared pet foods are 'ultra-processed'
  - There is some emerging evidence that ultra-processed foods might have detrimental effects on human health, including associations with cancer and obesity (Hall *et al.*, 2019; Schnabel *et al.*, 2019), but further work is required to determine the reasons for such associations
  - Commercially manufactured pet foods are not equivalent to ultra-processed foods for human consumption because they are designed to be complete and balanced when fed to meet maintenance energy requirements.
- Product recalls
  - Although a handful of products each year will be recalled (as with many human food products), the threat of imbalance or deficiency with commercially manufactured diets is significantly less compared with either home-prepared cooked or raw meat-based diets. Truly toxic components in pet foods have been found in only extremely rare cases.

- Additives and preservatives
  - The preservatives used to preserve pet foods and additives, as with all other ingredients, have until recently been under the strict control of the European Commission (EC); now that the UK has left the European Union (EU), new standards in accordance with the EC are being developed. The inclusion of preservatives in commercially manufactured foods adds to the convenience of storage by means of a reasonable shelf life. Additives also include vitamins and minerals, which make these diets complete and balanced.
- Damage to nutrients during the cooking process
  - Although some damage may occur during cooking, especially to proteins, the manufacturing process means that any deficiency is accounted for, and adjustments are made so a complete and balanced diet is still delivered.
- Rapid spoiling of wet food
  - Due to the high moisture content, wet food can start to spoil after about 30 minutes when left out at room temperature.
- Compliance issues
  - As with all diets, owner compliance will vary. Commercially manufactured diets should be correctly balanced; however, this will not remain the case if significant amounts of other food is also fed. Problems may also arise if the diet is fed in excess, as this can contribute to pet obesity (see Chapter 15). Adherence to the manufacturer's feeding guidelines is therefore recommended to prevent under- or overfeeding. However, it should be noted that there is considerable variation in the number of calories required by each individual pet. Food should be correctly portioned out each day (e.g. using digital scales). Treats and snacks unbalance the diet and add calories, which are not always accounted for in the daily feeding amount.

Safety measures when feeding commercially manufactured diets

In the UK and abroad, no matter what the diet, the form that it comes in or the scale of production, commercially manufactured diets must meet basic standards and criteria for production, packaging, formula reliability and pathogen control. More than 50 individual pieces of EU legislation govern the production of commercially manufactured diets (Food Standards Agency, 2017). Foods should:

- Be of a high quality
- Be free from pathogens
- Deliver complete and balanced nutrition.

Occasional failures in pathogen control procedures have been documented in a small number of cases, including:

- *Salmonella* spp. – found in uncooked commercially manufactured diets (Food Standards Agency, 2018a, 2019b)
- *Listeria* – found in uncooked commercially manufactured diets (Food Standards Agency, 2019a)
- *Mycobacterium bovis* – found in uncooked commercially manufactured cat food (O'Halloran *et al.*, 2019).

Occasional formulation errors (where nutrients have not been correctly balanced) have been recorded, including:

- Low thiamine concentrations – dry cat food (Pet Food Manufacturers' Association, 2015)
- Excess vitamin D – canned food (Food Standards Agency, 2018b; Hill's Pet Nutrition, 2019).

Very occasionally, fatal toxic components have been found including melamine contamination of a large number of commercially manufactured diets in North America in 2007 (US Food and Drug Administration, 2007). No pet foods were affected outside of North America. Compared with other diet types (e.g. home-prepared cooked diets or raw meat-based diets), pathogenic infection and nutritional imbalances are far less frequent, especially when considering the number of pets fed this type of diet annually. It is estimated that 95% of dog owners and 98% of cat owners feed their pet a commercially manufactured diet as part of or as the whole diet (PDSA, 2019).

Considerations for feeding commercially manufactured diets

Healthy dogs and cats

Commercially manufactured diets are complete and balanced and, provided that the amount fed is as per the guidelines specified on the packaging, can be a healthy option for dogs and cats.

Dogs and cats with various diseases

Many different diseases have specific nutritional requirements and there is dietetic food available to manage pets with such conditions and their requirements. Optimal nutrition during a disease state may be pivotal to the survival of the individual.

Conclusion

Feeding a commercially manufactured diet can offer optimal nutrition to patients without high costs, with low pathogen risk and with nutritional assurance. However, care should be taken, particularly with dry food, to ensure it is not fed in excess.

References and further reading

Allan FJ, Pfeiffer DU, Jones BR, Esslemont DHB and Wiseman MS (2000) A cross-sectional study of risk factors for obesity in cats. *Preventative Veterinary Medicine* **46**, 183–196

Axelsson E, Ratnakumar A, Arendt ML *et al.* (2013) The genomic signature of dog domestication reveals adaptation to a starch rich diet. *Nature* **495**, 360–364

Beynen AC (2018) Wet food and calorie intake by cats. *Creature Companion* **38**, 40

Biourge V (2004) Diagnosis of adverse reactions to food in dogs: efficacy of a soy-isolate hydrolyzate-based diet. *Journal of Nutrition* **134**, 2062S–2064S

Bissot T, Servet E, Vidal S *et al.* (2009) Novel dietary strategies can improve the outcome of weight loss programmes in obese client-owned cats. *Journal of Feline Medicine and Surgery* **12**, 104–112

Carciofi AC, Bazolli RS, Zanni A, Kihara LRL and Prada F (2005) Influence of water content and the digestibility of pet foods on the water balance of cats. *Brazilian Journal of Veterinary Research and Animal Science* **42**, 429–434

Case LP (2010) Chronic renal failure. In: *Canine and Feline Nutrition, 3rd edn*, ed. L Case *et al.*, pp. 418–420. Mosby Elsevier, Philadelphia

Case LP, Carey DP, Hirakawa DA and Daristotle L (2000) *Canine and Feline Nutrition, 2nd edn.* Mosby Elsevier, Philadelphia

Commission Regulation (EU) 1334/2008 of the European Parliament and Council (2008) *On flavourings and certain food ingredients with flavouring properties for use in and on foods and amending Council Regulation (EEC) No. 1601/91, Regulations (EC) No. 2232/96 and (EC) No. 110/2008 and Directive 2000/13/EC.* [Available from: https://eur-lex.europa.eu/legal-content/EN/TXT/?qid=1585739671020&uri=CELEX:32008R1334]

Commission Regulation (EU) 2020/354 (2020) *Establishing a list of intended uses of feed intended for particular nutritional purposes and repealing Directive 2008/38/EC.* [Available from: https://eur-lex.europa.eu/legal-content/EN/TXT/?uri=CELEX:32020R0354]

FEDIAF (2024) *Nutritional guidelines for complete and complementary pet food in cats and dogs.* [Available from: https://europeanpetfood.org/wp-content/uploads/2024/09/FEDIAF-Nutritional-Guidelines_2024.pdf]

Food Standards Agency (2017) *Business Guidance – Pet Food.* [Available from: www.food.gov.uk/business-guidance/pet-food]

Food Standards Agency (2018a) *Avondale Pet Foods Ltd recalls Just Natural Chicken and Tripe because Salmonella has been found in the produce.* [Available from: www.food.gov.uk/news-alerts/alert/fsa-prin-71-2018]

Food Standards Agency (2018b) *Sainsbury's recalls a range of its pet food pouch selections due to high levels of vitamin D.* [Available from: www.food.gov.uk/news-alerts/alert/fsa-prin-25-2018]

Food Standards Agency (2019a) *Raw Treat Pet Food Ltd recalls frozen raw beef, chicken, lamb, and chicken and tripe pet food due to the presence of Listeria monocytogenes.* [Available from: www.food.gov.uk/news-alerts/alert/fsa-prin-36-2019]aA

Food Standards Agency (2019b) *Raw Treat Pet Food Ltd recalls varieties of frozen raw pet food due to the presence of Salmonella.* [Available from: www.food.gov.uk/news-alerts/alert/fsa-prin-38-]

German AJ, Holden SL, Bissot T, Morris PJ and Biourge V (2010) A high protein, high fibre diet improves weight loss in obese dogs. *The Veterinary Journal* **183**, 294–297

Hall KD, Ayuketah A, Brychta R *et al.* (2019) Ultra-processed diets cause excess calorie intake and weight gain: an inpatient randomized controlled trial of *ad libitum* food intake. *Cell Metabolism* **30**, 1–11

Hill's Pet Nutrition (2019) *Important voluntary product recall information.* [Available from www.hillspet.co.uk/productlist]

Jackson OF and Tovey JD (1977) Water balance studies in domestic cats. *Feline Practice* **7(4)**, 30–33

Kendall PT and Holme DW (1982) Studies on digestibility of soya bean products, cereal, cereal and plant by products in the diet of dogs. *Journal of the Science of Food and Agriculture* **33**, 813–820

Morris GJ, Trudell J and Pencovic T (1977) Carbohydrate digestion by the domestic cat (*Felis catus*). *British Journal of Nutrition* **37(3)**, 365–373

O'Halloran C, Ioannidi O, Reed N *et al.* (2019) Tuberculosis due to *Mycobacterium bovis* in pet cats associated with feeding a commercial raw food diet. *Journal of Feline Medicine and Surgery* **21(8)**, 667–681

Öhlund M, Palmgren M and Holst BS (2018) Overweight in adult cats: a cross-sectional study. *Acta Veterinaria Scandinavica* **60**, 5

PDSA (2019) *PDSA Animal Wellbeing Report (PAW) Report.* [Available from: www.pdsa.org.uk/media/7420/2019-paw-report_downloadable.pdf]

Pet Food Manufacturers' Association (2015) *Pets at Home recall.* [Available from: www.pfma.org.uk/news/pets-at-home-recall]

Polzin D (2019) *International Renal Interest Society – Diets for Cats with Chronic Kidney Disease (CKD).* [Available from: http://www.iris-kidney.com/education/protein_restriction_feline_ckd.html]

Roberts MT, Bermingham EN, Cave NJ *et al.* (2018) Macronutrient intake of dogs: self-selecting diets varying in composition offered *ad libitum*. *Journal of Animal Physiology and Animal Nutrition* **102**, 568–575

Robertson ID (1999) The influence of diet and other factors on owner-perceived obesity in privately owned cats from metropolitan Perth, Western Australia. *Preventative Veterinary Medicine* **40** 75–85

Russell K, Sabin R, Holt S, Bradley R and Harper EJ (2000) Influence of feeding regimen on body condition in the cat. *Journal of Small Animal Practice* **41**, 12–17

Schnabel L, Kesse-Guyot E, Allès B *et al.* (2019) Association between ultra-processed food consumption and risk of mortality among middle-aged adults in France. *Journal of the American Medical Association: Internal Medicine* **179(4)**, 490–498

Tarttelin MF (1987) Feline struvite urolithiasis: factors affecting urine pH may be more important than magnesium levels in food. *Veterinary Record* **121(10)**, 227–30

US Food and Drug Administration (2007) *Melamine Pet Food Recall.* [Available from: www.fda.gov/animal-veterinary/recallswithdrawals/melamine-pet-food-recall-frequently-asked-questions]

van Bree FPJ, Bokken GCAM, Mineur R *et al.* (2018) Zoonotic bacteria and parasites found in raw meat-based diets for cats and dogs. *Veterinary Record* **182(2)**, 50

Wall M, Cave NJ and Vallee E (2019) Owner and cat-related risk factors for feline overweight or obesity. *Frontiers in Veterinary Science* **19(6)**, 266

Weber M, Bissot T, Servet E *et al.* (2007) A high-protein, high-fiber diet designed for weight loss improves satiety in dogs. *Journal of Veterinary Internal Medicine* **21**, 1203–1208

Useful websites

World Small Animal Veterinary Association (WSAVA):

- Global Nutrition Toolkit
  https://wsava.org/wp-content/uploads/2020/01/WSAVA-Global-Nutrition-Toolkit-English.pdf
- Interpreting Food Labels
  http://www.wsava.org/wp-content/uploads/2020/01/Nutrition-Label-EU-16_9.pdf

Online extras

This chapter includes:

- A client information leaflet that is available to download and print from the BSAVA Library

Access via QR code or: bsavalibrary.com/nutrition_3

Grain-free diets

4

Grain-free diets have increased in popularity in recent years with most brands of pet food now offering a grain-free option to satisfy demand. However, recent evidence has come to light that the inclusion of some ingredients in large amounts in the diet of dogs and cats could be causing detrimental health effects in some instances. Grain-free diets typically do not contain the following ingredients:

- Wheat (Figure 4.1a)
- Barley
- Rice
- Maize (Figure 4.1b)
- Sorghum (Figure 4.1c)
- Spelt
- Bulgar
- Farro
- Millet (Figure 4.1d)
- Oats
- Rye
- Malt
- Brewer's yeast
- Wheat starch
- Triticale (a wheat/rye hybrid).

It should be noted that grains contain different types of gluten, some of which may not be of concern, even for those pets known to have an adverse food reaction to glutens (such adverse reactions are uncommon). However, a blanket approach is often taken and all grains are excluded from the diet, meaning that a number of other nutrients that grains deliver are also restricted when there may be no requirement to do so (Pezzali et al., 2020).

Grains can be a useful source of protein, essential fatty acids, vitamins, minerals and fibre. Digestibility is typically high when included in pet foods (Kendall and Holme, 1982). Cooked whole grains may be harder to digest compared with meat-based products. Dogs as a species are nutritionally omnivorous and are fully equipped to extract nutrients from grain sources in their diets. Cats, while being obligate carnivores (i.e. requiring meat, poultry or fish in their diet), also have the ability to digest and obtain nutrients from grains (Morris et al., 1977).

There are concerns that grains are not part of a 'natural' diet for dogs and cats based on their wild ancestors; however, the European Pet Food Industry Federation (FEDIAF) guidance for the term 'natural' states that the term should be used only to describe substances in pet food (i.e. derived from plants, animals, microorganisms or minerals) to which nothing has been added, and which have been subjected to only physical processing to make them suitable for pet food production whilst maintaining their natural composition.

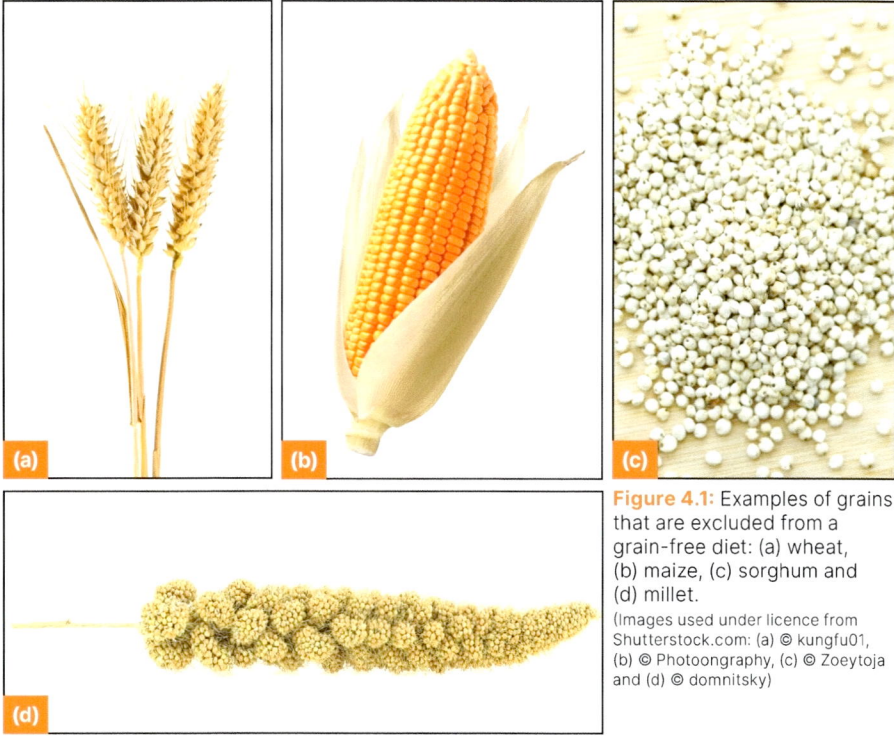

Figure 4.1: Examples of grains that are excluded from a grain-free diet: (a) wheat, (b) maize, (c) sorghum and (d) millet.

(Images used under licence from Shutterstock.com: (a) © kungfu01, (b) © Photoongraphy, (c) © Zoeytoja and (d) © domnitsky)

In addition, some owners believe that grain-free diets are a 'healthier option' for their pet (Tufts-Cumming School of Veterinary Medicine Nutrition Service, 2016). There is, however, limited evidence that gluten is 'unhealthy' or makes pets unwell, except in rare cases of adverse food reactions (Batt *et al.*, 1982) (see Chapter 14). To compound the confusion, a commonly held misperception is that diets that are grain-free are also carbohydrate-free (which is desirable for some pet owners), which is not necessarily the case. Other carbohydrate sources (e.g. potato) are frequently used in grain-free diets.

Types of grain-free diet

Grain-free diets are now commercially produced by many pet food manufacturers in the United Kingdom (UK) in a wet or dry form. Ideally, such diets should be created by professional formulators trained in the commercial formulation of pet foods, in consultation with an appropriately qualified individual (see Chapter 1).

For those owners that prefer home-prepared diets, it is possible for a grain-free diet to be formulated but it is highly recommended that the recipe be designed, overseen or approved by an appropriately qualified individual. Provided that the recipe and supplement recommendations are followed carefully, these can provide a complete and balanced nutritional diet.

Advantages of feeding a grain-free diet

There are evidence-based advantages for feeding a grain-free diet in some instances. They are often used during food elimination trials where an adverse reaction is being investigated, particularly in cases of skin disease or gastrointestinal signs (see Chapter 14). The main concern with regards to feeding grains relates to a perceived risk of an allergy to glutens and gliadins (Case *et al.*, 2000); however, the foods most commonly associated with adverse food reactions in dogs and cats are beef, soya and dairy products (August, 1985; Hodgkins, 1991; Harvey, 1993). Dietary gluten elimination improves clinical signs associated with paroxysmal gluten-sensitive dyskinesia, a neurological disorder that mainly affects Border Terriers (Lowrie *et al.*, 2015). Clinical signs range from mild abnormal movement of one limb affecting function or coordination, to severe, where dogs collapse and abnormal movement affects the whole body.

Disadvantages of feeding a grain-free diet

Although both dogs and cats can seemingly do well on grain-free diets, there have been some reports of health problems developing, most notably dilated cardiomyopathy (DCM) in dogs (Freeman *et al.*, 2018) (Figure 4.2). The exact causal factors and pathogenetic mechanisms remain unclear, but questions have arisen as to whether the absence of grains is the problem. However, since some grain-free diets are made by established food companies, it is possible that wider formulation problems are the cause. It was found that the same ingredients repeatedly appeared listed in the diets of affected dogs, and since many of the affected dogs improved after switching to a non-grain-free diet, this led to the suspicion that the diet was the cause. Further work is required to improve the understanding of the pathophysiology and to determine the risks; caution is advised when using a grain-free diet in breeds prone to DCM (e.g. Dobermanns) and known cases of DCM. Should a grain-free diet be required for the pet (e.g. in case of adverse reaction to food), products that have undergone feeding trials to ensure nutritional adequacy would be recommended.

Safety measures when feeding grain-free diets

Basic health and safety should be observed when buying and feeding commercially produced grain-free diets (see Chapter 1). For information on safety measures that should be observed when handling home-prepared diets, see Chapter 5.

Considerations for feeding grain-free diets

Healthy dogs and cats

To feed a grain-free diet correctly, an appropriate product should be selected that has been specifically formulated for the desired life stage. If the grain-free diet is home-prepared, an appropriately qualified individual should be consulted (see Chapter 1) or approved recipes and supplements fed. This is especially important if the pet is young or senior in years.

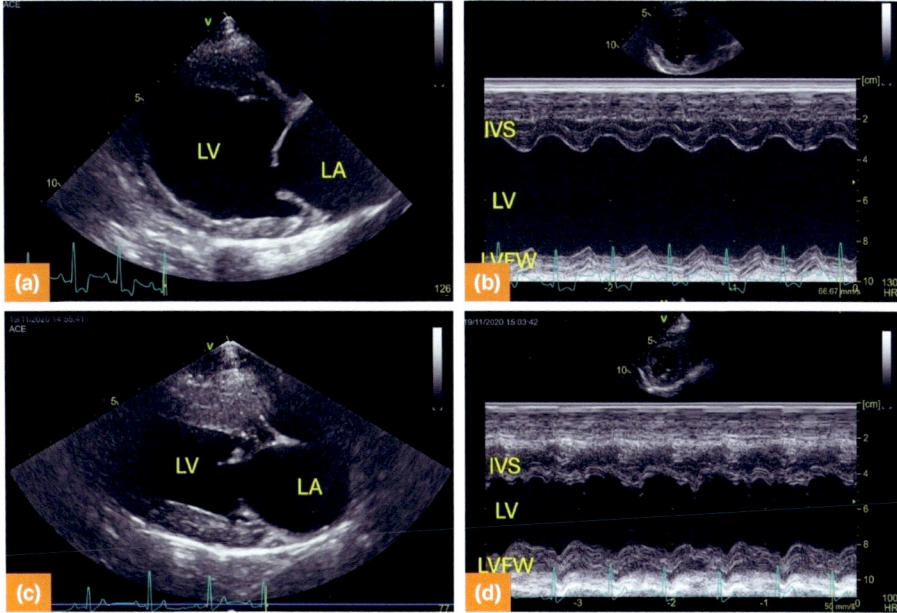

Figure 4.2: Echocardiograms from a Labrador Retriever with dilated cardiomyopathy (DCM). The patient was being fed a grain-free diet and presented with congestive heart failure. (a, c) Right parasternal four-chamber views and (b, d) left ventricular M-mode views at the level of the chordae tendinae. (a) Left atrial and left ventricular dilatation are present. Note also the relatively thin left ventricular walls. (b) The pump function of the left ventricle was poor in real-time. Following a change in diet, including taurine supplementation, and the administration of conventional cardiac medications, such as furosemide, pimobendan, benazepril and spironolactone, (c) less dilatation was observed in the left ventricle and left atrium, and (d) there was improved pump function. IVS = interventricular septum; LA = left atrium; LV = left ventricle; LVFW = left ventricular free wall.
(© Jo Dukes-McEwan, University of Liverpool)

Dogs and cats with various diseases
Grain-free diets are essential only in a minority of cases. Key examples include adverse reactions to food proved to be caused by gluten (e.g. as determined by an exclusion diet trial). Some grain-free diets might be detrimental to pets that do not require them.

Conclusion
Feeding grain-free diets has become increasingly popular in recent years, so it is important that veterinary professionals are aware of available options, as well as the pros and cons when advising owners of the best diet to feed their pet. Decisions will often be made 'on balance' for the individual. Advice based on good evidence should be given and any recommendation must ensure that the minimum requirements are met to ensure complete and balanced nutrition.

References and further reading

August JR (1985) Dietary hypersensitivity in dogs: cutaneous manifestations, diagnosis and management. *Compendium on Continuing Education for the Practicing Veterinarian* **7**, 469–477

Batt RM, Carter MW and McLean L (1982) Morphological and biochemical studies of a naturally occurring enteropathy in the Irish setter dog: comparison with coeliac disease in man. *Research in Veterinary Science* **37(3)**, 339–346

Case LP, Carey DP, Hirakawa DA and Daristotle L (2000) *Canine and Feline Nutrition, 2nd edn.* Mosby Elsevier, Philadelphia

Freeman LM, Stern JA, Fries R, Adin DB and Rush JE (2018) Diet-associated dilated cardiomyopathy in dogs: what do we know? *Journal of the American Veterinary Medical Association* **253(11)**, 1390–1394

Harvey RG (1993) Food allergy and dietary intolerance in dogs: a report of 25 cases. *Journal of Small Animal Practice* **34**, 175–179

Hodgkins E (1991) Food allergy in cats: considerations, diagnosis and management. *Pet Vet* **24**, 8

Jeffers JG, Shanley and Meyer EK (1991) Diagnostic testing of dogs for food hypersensitivity. *Journal of the American Veterinary Medical Association* **198**, 245–250

Kendall PT and Holme DW (1982) Studies on the digestibility of soya bean products, cereals, cereal and plant by-products in the diets of dogs. *Journal of the Science of Food and Agriculture* **33**, 813–820

Lowrie M, Garden OA, Hadjivassiliou M *et al.* (2015) The clinical and serological effect of a gluten-free diet in Border Terriers with epileptoid cramping syndrome. *Journal of Veterinary Internal Medicine* **29(6)**, 1564–1569

Morris GJ, Trudell J and Pencovic T (1977) Carbohydrate digestion by the domestic cat (*Felis catus*). *British Journal of Nutrition* **37(3)**, 365–373

Pezzali JG, Acuff HL, Henry W *et al.* (2020) Effects of different carbohydrate sources on taurine status in healthy Beagle dogs. *Journal of Animal Science* **98(2)**, 1–9

Tufts-Cumming School of Veterinary Medicine Nutrition Service (2016) *Grain-free diets – big on marketing, small on truth.* [Available from: https://vetnutrition.tufts.edu/2016/06/grain-free-diets-big-on-marketing-small-on-truth/.]

Online extras

This chapter includes:

- A client information leaflet that is available to download and print from the BSAVA Library

Access via QR code or: bsavalibrary.com/nutrition_4

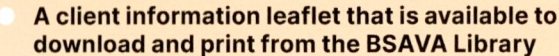

Home-prepared cooked diets

5

Home-prepared cooked diets comprise cooked ingredients, with the exception of some uncooked vegetables, fruits and nuts (Figure 5.1). Similar to raw meat-based diets, home-prepared cooked diets contain ingredients that can be easily purchased and, with the exception of some dairy products and oils, have undergone limited processing.

Depending on the home-prepared cooked diet type, the following specific ingredients may be included:

- Meat
- Fish
- Poultry
- Green or yellow vegetables
- Root vegetables
- Eggs
- Dairy products
- Cereals
- Oils
- Nuts
- Seeds
- Fruits.

Types of home-prepared cooked diet

Home-prepared cooked diet recipes are widely available from sources such as books, magazines and the internet. They may also be produced by an appropriately qualified individual (see Chapter 1). However, caution is needed because not all recipes will deliver complete and balanced nutrition. Pet owners should be encouraged to contact an appropriately qualified individual to have their recipe assessed to make sure it is complete and balanced. Some home-prepared cooked diets are designed to be fed alongside a nutritional supplement and the feeding guidelines should be clearly stated on the recipe. Furthermore, there are some owners that may opt to feed their pet according to its preferences, without using a recipe.

> In a study assessing 200 different home-prepared cooked diet recipes that were **not** created by an appropriately qualified person, 94% of the diets had a deficiency of one essential nutrient and 84% of the diets had a deficiency of more than one essential nutrient (Fell, 2013).

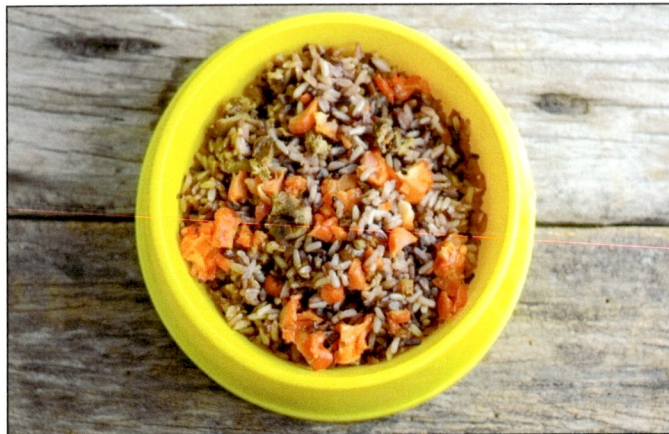

Figure 5.1: Example of a home-prepared cooked pet food containing cooked brown rice, cooked chicken and liver and cooked carrot.
(Image used under licence from Shutterstock.com: © aukarawatcyber)

Advantages of feeding a home-prepared cooked diet

- Used in diet trials short-term
  - It can be easier to design an appropriate short-term elimination trial if a home-prepared cooked diet is used. Trials typically last for 2–10 weeks and, if appropriately conducted, can be used for diagnosing adverse food reactions (see Chapter 14) (Jeffers *et al.*, 1991). If used for short periods of time, such diets need not be complete and balanced; however, if the diet successfully resolves the clinical signs of an adverse food reaction, it can be considered for long-term feeding, but only if it is then suitably balanced by an appropriately qualified individual (see Chapter 1).
- Used when there is no other suitable diet
  - Where there is a **proven** adverse reaction to food and no suitable commercially produced diet is available, a home-prepared cooked diet can be used provided it has been created by an appropriately qualified individual and is safe for long-term use
  - In cases where concurrent disease is present alongside an adverse reaction to food, home-prepared cooked diets can be tailored to meet the needs of the individual pet; for example, for patients with renal disease, protein and phosphorus restriction is vital (Ross *et al.*, 1982; Finco *et al.*, 1992) (see Chapter 19).
- Improved palatability
  - Depending on the formulation, home-prepared cooked diets often have a greater moisture content and may also contain more fat and protein. Foods that the pet likes are generally chosen. Improved palatability is therefore expected. This may be an advantage for picky eaters but a disadvantage for pets prone to obesity.
- The diet is cooked *versus* a raw meat-based diet
  - The cooking of ingredients in home-prepared cooked diets reduces the risk of pathogenic infection compared with feeding diets that are uncooked.
- A more 'natural' food
  - Guidance for the term 'natural' is that it must be obtained exclusively (or at least 95%) from the source material (e.g. of vegetable or animal origin). This is not an official or regulated definition; therefore, depending on the ingredients used, commercially manufactured diets can also be defined as 'natural' in accordance with the guidance (Commission Regulation, 2008).

- Ultra-processed content
  - Although there is some emerging evidence that ultra-processed foods may be of concern to humans, further work in this area is needed (Schnabel *et al.*, 2019). In general, pet foods are not considered to be ultra-processed by the definitions used for human food.
- Can be carbohydrate/gluten/wheat free
  - A study has shown that over the many years of dog domestication, their dietary needs have changed and their digestive capabilities have adapted to accommodate living as companions (Axelson *et al.*, 2013). Unlike their ancestors, domesticated dogs can readily digest carbohydrates; 10 of the 36 genomic differences between these species are involved in carbohydrate digestion (Axelson *et al.*, 2013).
- Improved stool volume
  - A smaller stool volume would be expected if home-prepared cooked diets contain a lower fibre content than commercially prepared diets.
- Can be fed at all life stages
  - This will only be the case if the recipe was created by an appropriately qualified individual (see Chapter 1) and is appropriate for all life stages, including growth and reproduction.

Disadvantages of feeding a home-prepared cooked diet

- Cost
  - The cost of feeding a home-prepared cooked diet is significantly greater than other types of diet, especially commercially produced dry foods. Increased costs are due to sourcing ingredients and specific supplements that are essential for completing the nutritional profile of the diet. These costs are in addition to the cost of the diet formulation creation by an appropriately qualified individual (see Chapter 1). For large dog breeds, these costs may be prohibitive.
- Cooking and preparation time
  - Home-prepared cooked diets require the cooking of ingredients every 1–2 days. It takes significantly longer to prepare each meal than it would for pre-prepared foods, and many owners will find this commitment difficult to maintain. Even if batch-cooked and frozen, the meals still take time to thaw, reheat and cool compared with other diet types which can be ready in seconds.
- Pathogenic infection
  - Compared with feeding a raw meat-based diet, the risk from pathogens is less, making home-prepared cooked diets safer overall. However, care is still required when meals have been pre-prepared because incorrect cooking, cooling, thawing and reheating can result in bacterial growth, which may lead to a potential risk of food poisoning.
- Decreased digestibility
  - Although cooking can denature proteins, reducing their digestibility, this is only a minor effect and can be easily compensated without the pet having to consume the diet in excess to meet their nutritional needs. Cooking can also increase the digestibility of many other ingredients. Even though reduced digestibility is undesirable, the benefits of cooking the ingredients and avoiding pathogenesis are a significant advantage for both the pet's and owner's health.

- Compliance
  - As with any diet, the level of compliance from owners will vary. Given that it is harder to balance a home-prepared cooked diet, the margin for error may be smaller and so mistakes leading to deficiency are easier to make. It is important to impress on pet owners the need for excellent compliance while feeding a home-prepared cooked diet, to ensure that the diet being fed each day is complete and sufficiently balanced.

Example calculation for cost comparisons of diets

Species: Canine   **Age:** 8 years old   **Weight:** 12 kg

Food preference:
Fish (cod) and brown rice

Cost of diet formulation:
£185
For the formulation to be created by an appropriately qualified individual.
Prices may vary.

Cost of diet ingredients:
£177 per month
Price based on sourcing ingredients from high street supermarkets and using unbranded or own-branded items.

Cost of supplement:
£26.69 per month

Cost of shipping:
£66.02 one off price per shipment

Total cost of feeding the home-prepared cooked diet:
£454.71 for the first month, £203.69 per month thereafter

Comparative cost of feeding a commercially produced wet food:
£37.20 per month.
Price based on Pedigree® Adult complete dog food tins.

Comparative costs of feeding a commercially produced dry food:
£8.40 per month.
Price based on Pedigree® Adult complete dry food.

Excess or deficiency in the diet

When feeding a home-prepared cooked diet, it is difficult for the owner to ensure that what they are feeding is a complete and balanced diet for their pet. Research studies have assessed the nutritional adequacy of home-prepared cooked diets. Two such studies looking at 94 commonly available recipes for homemade diets (both cooked and uncooked) for pets with medical conditions found them all to be inadequate (Heinze *et al.*, 2012; Larsen *et al.*, 2012). A third study of 200 different recipes for maintenance diets for dogs, found that 95% were deficient in at least one essential element and 84% had multiple deficiencies (Stockman *et al.*, 2013).

Clinical signs associated with conditions that are caused by feeding an unbalanced diet can take a considerable period of time to appear. At this point the damage may be irreversible. Deficiencies of certain nutrients include insufficient calcium in the diet, which occurs when an all-meat, table-scrap or all organ meat diet is fed. These diets, being very low in calcium, cause hypocalcaemia resulting in nutritional secondary hyperparathyroidism (Figure 5.2). This is a very painful condition leading to significant bone loss through demineralization and multiple pathological bone fractures (Bennett, 1976; Hintz and Schryver, 1987).

Although there are no published studies on prevalence, the risk of nutrient deficiencies causing overt clinical signs in otherwise healthy adult dogs and cats appears to be rare. However, such deficiencies are more frequently reported in growing animals. As a result, caution should be exercised when feeding such diets to animals

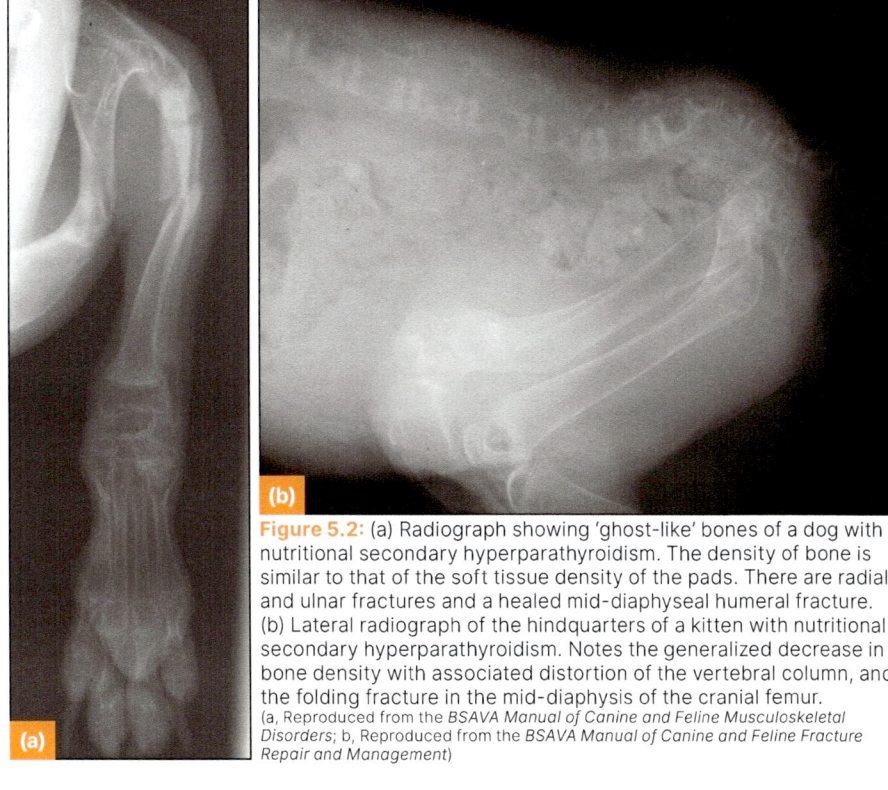

Figure 5.2: (a) Radiograph showing 'ghost-like' bones of a dog with nutritional secondary hyperparathyroidism. The density of bone is similar to that of the soft tissue density of the pads. There are radial and ulnar fractures and a healed mid-diaphyseal humeral fracture. (b) Lateral radiograph of the hindquarters of a kitten with nutritional secondary hyperparathyroidism. Notes the generalized decrease in bone density with associated distortion of the vertebral column, and the folding fracture in the mid-diaphysis of the cranial femur.
(a, Reproduced from the *BSAVA Manual of Canine and Feline Musculoskeletal Disorders*; b, Reproduced from the *BSAVA Manual of Canine and Feline Fracture Repair and Management*)

that have not yet reached skeletal maturity. It should also be noted that appropriate feeding trials are performed for good quality commercial diets. Whereas, when a home-prepared cooked diet is provided, the food trial is essentially being performed on the owner's pet. Nutrient interactions and bioavailability cannot be determined for home-prepared cooked diets. In addition, if a vitamin supplement is added to the recipe prior to cooking, many of the vitamins can be destroyed by the cooking process.

Safety measures when feeding home-prepared cooked diets

Hygiene

Basic hygiene is essential for the safe feeding of a home-prepared cooked diet to prevent pathogen infection (see Chapter 1).

Cooling, storing and reheating a home-prepared cooked diet

To prevent bacterial growth and subsequent food poisoning, care should be taken when cooling cooked foods. Uneaten cooked meals can be stored and reheated at a later date, provided that:

- Food is cooled to room temperature completely before it is covered and refrigerated
- Food is not cooled in the refrigerator because this can increase the temperature inside, increasing risk of spoilage of other foods
- Food is stored in a sealed container in either the refrigerator or freezer
- When needed, food must be reheated only once
- On reheating, food should be piping hot throughout and allowed to cool to an edible temperature before being fed to the pet.

Considerations for feeding home-prepared cooked diets

To feed a home-prepared cooked diet correctly for any stage of life, or for pets who have a disease requiring nutritional alteration, an appropriately qualified individual should be consulted and only approved recipes and supplements fed. This is especially important if the pet is young (i.e. still growing) or intended to be involved in reproduction (see Chapter 9), when nutritional requirements differ from those of an adult.

Feeding home-prepared cooked diets in a hospital environment

As more patients are being fed home-prepared cooked diets, it is important to consider the affect that this may have in a veterinary hospital setting (see Chapter 12). Preparing food as the owner would at home is often impractical and discussion with the owner regarding alternatives will be necessary. Owners may need or want to cook and bring food in daily for their pet. Each veterinary practice might wish to create and enforce their own policy with regards to this, as the sources of ingredients and hygiene during preparation cannot be guaranteed. Pathogen risk is low but, as with any food, basic hygiene rules should apply. There should be no need to isolate a patient fed a home-prepared cooked diet on this basis alone, unlike those fed a raw meat-based diet (see Chapter 6) where the risk of pathogenic infection to other patients and staff is higher.

Conclusion

It is important that veterinary professionals first educate themselves about the available options, and then consider all the pros and cons when advising owners of the best diet to feed their pet. Decisions will often be made 'on balance' for the individual. Advice based on good evidence, wherever available, should be given each time, and any recommendation must ensure that minimum nutritional requirements are met. In such cases, home-prepared cooked diets can provide complete, balanced and safe nutrition.

References and further reading

Arthurs G, Brown G and Pettitt R (2018) *BSAVA Manual of Canine and Feline Musculoskeletal Disorders, 2nd edn.* BSAVA Publications, Gloucester

August JR (1985) Dietary hypersensitivity in dogs: cutaneous manifestations, diagnosis and management. *Compendium on Continuing Education for the Practicing Veterinarian* **7**, 469–477

Axelson E, Ratnakumar A, Arendt ML *et al.* (2013) The genomic signature of dog domestication reveals adaptation to a starch rich diet. *Nature* **495**, 360–364

Bennett D (1976) Nutrition and bone disease in dogs and cats. *Veterinary Record* **98**, 313–320

Commission Regulation (EU) 1334/2008 of the European Parliament and Council (2008) *On flavourings and certain food ingredients with flavouring properties for use in and on foods and amending Council Regulation (EEC) No. 1601/91, Regulations (EC) No. 2232/96 and (EC) No. 110/2008 and Directive 2000/13/EC.* [Available from: https://eur-lex.europa.eu/legal-content/EN/TXT/?qid=1585739671020&uri=CELEX:32008R1334]

Fell A (2013) *Homemade dog food recipes can be risky business, study finds.* [Available from: https://www.ucdavis.edu/news/homemade-dog-food-recipes-can-be-risky-business-study-finds/]

Finco DR, Brown SA, Crowell WA *et al.* (1992) Effects of dietary phosphorus and protein in dogs with chronic renal failure. *American Journal of Veterinary Research* **53(12)**, 2264–2271

Gemmill TJ and Clements DN (2016) *BSAVA Manual of Canine and Feline Fracture Repair and Management, 2nd edn.* BSAVA Publications, Gloucester

Harvey RG (1993) Food allergy and dietary intolerance in dogs: a report of 25 cases. *Journal of Small Animal Practice* **34**, 175–179

Heinze CR, Gomez FC and Freeman LM (2012) Assessment of commercial diets and recipes for home prepared diets recommended for dogs with cancer. *Journal of the American Veterinary Medical Association* **241**, 1453–1460

Hintz HF and Schryver HF (1987) Nutrition and bone development in dogs. *European Journal of Companion Animal Practice* **1**, 44–47

Hodgkins E (1991) Food allergy in cats: considerations, diagnosis and management. *Pet Vet* **24**, 8

Jeffers JG, Shanley and Meyer EK (1991) Diagnostic testing of dogs for food hypersensitivity. *Journal of the American Veterinary Medical Association* **198**, 245–250

Larsen JA, Parks EM, Heinze CR and Fascetti AJ (2012) Evaluation of recipes for home prepared diets for dogs and cats with chronic kidney disease. *Journal of the American Veterinary Medical Association* **240**, 532–538

Morris GJ, Trudell J and Pencovic T (1977) Carbohydrate digestion by the domestic cat (*Felis catus*). *British Journal of Nutrition* **37(3)**, 365–373

Ross LA, Finco DR and Crowell WA (1982) Effect of phosphorus restriction on the kidneys of cats with reduced renal mass. *American Journal of Veterinary Research* **43(6)**, 1023–1026

Schnabel L, Kesse-Guyot E, Allès B *et al.* (2019) Association between ultra-processed food consumption and risk of mortality among middle-aged adults in France. *Journal of the American Medical Association: Internal Medicine* **179(4)**, 490–498

Stockman J, Fascetti AJ, Kass PH and Larsen JA (2013) Evaluation of recipes of home-prepared maintenance diets for dogs. *Journal of the American Veterinary Medical Association* **242**, 1500–1505

Online extras

This chapter includes:

- A client information leaflet that is available to download and print from the BSAVA Library

Access via QR code or: bsavalibrary.com/nutrition_5

Raw meat-based diets | 6

Raw meat-based diets (RMBDs) (also known as 'biologically appropriate raw food' (BARF) diets) are becoming increasingly popular with owners. Veterinary professionals need to provide guidance about the advantages and disadvantages of such foods. RMBDs predominately comprise a wide variety of uncooked ingredients including:

- Meat
- Fish
- Poultry
- Bones
- Meat by-products (offal)
- Unpasteurized milk
- Uncooked egg
- Fruit and vegetables
- Nuts and seeds
- Oils
- Cereals.

Types of raw meat-based diet

The following types of RMBD are available:

- Commercially manufactured. Within this category, there are various options, including:
  - Fresh (Figure 6.1a)
  - Frozen (Figure 6.1b)
  - Freeze-dried (Figure 6.1c)
  - Carbohydrate premix with a raw protein source
  - Kibble with freeze-dried raw pieces
  - Diets with a raw-meat coating.
- Home-prepared:
  - Feeding to a recipe
  - No recipe: any available food is fed (not recommended).
- Prey-model – whole animal carcasses are fed.

Some commercially prepared RMBD recipes are created by professional formulators trained in the commercial formulation of pet foods, in consultation with an appropriately qualified individual (see Chapter 1). In the case of home-prepared raw diets, recipes may not be complete and balanced; therefore, it is recommended that owners consult an appropriately qualified individual to design a recipe before feeding a RMBD to their pet.

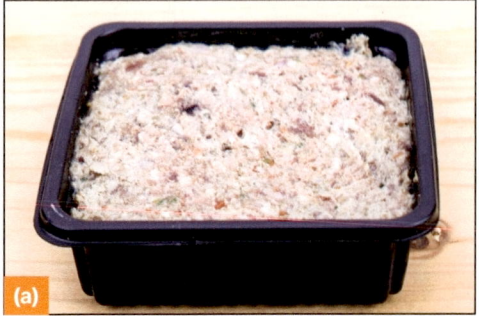

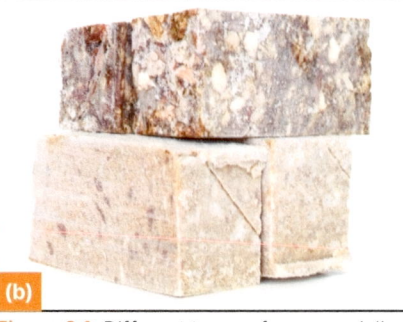

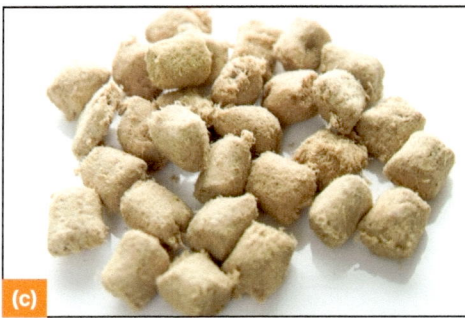

Figure 6.1: Different types of commercially available raw dog and cat food: (a) fresh mince, (b) frozen blocks and (c) freeze-dried pellets.
(Images used under the licence from Shutterstock.com: (a) © ThamKC, (b) © sophiecat and (c) © Anna Hoychuk)

Advantages of feeding a raw meat-based diet

Currently, there are insufficient published scientific studies confirming many of the suggested benefits of RMBDs, although there is emerging evidence to support some claims. The suggested benefits include:

- Dental benefits from chewing raw bones with meat
  - There is limited evidence to suggest that the texture of chewing raw bones with meat could be beneficial for dental calculus reduction. However, there is no evidence that it improves oral health or prevents plaque, periodontitis or tooth loss (Marx *et al.*, 2016). Bones, raw or cooked, can also pose a risk of dental fractures, oesophageal obstructions and foreign bodies.
- Improved coat quality (Billinghurst, 1993)
  - It has been suggested that this might be the result of feeding a diet with an increased fat content. Any benefits of feeding a high fat diet should be balanced against potential risks (e.g. obesity and pancreatitis).
- Improved digestibility
  - This is partially true; RMBDs are typically more digestible than dry proprietary food, but not necessarily wet proprietary food (Freeman *et al.*, 2013). Digestibility also depends on the ingredients and specific nutrients contained within the diet (Hamper *et al.*, 2016).
- Improved palatability
  - Food with a greater moisture content will be more palatable to some dogs and high protein diets are more palatable for cats. This may be an advantage for picky eaters but could be a disadvantage for pets prone to obesity.

- A more 'natural' food
  - Guidance for the term 'natural' is that it must be obtained exclusively (or at least 95%) from the source material (e.g. vegetable or animal origin). This is not an official or regulated definition; therefore, depending on the ingredients used, commercially manufactured diets can also be defined as 'natural' in accordance with the above guidance (Commission Regulation, 2008).
- More appropriate diet for dogs
  - As wolves are similar to dogs, it has been suggested that the sort of diet they consume may be more appropriate for dogs than other types of diet (e.g. processed kibble or canned food). However, a study has shown that over the many years of dog domestication, their dietary requirements have changed and their digestive capabilities have adapted to accommodate living as companions (Axelsson *et al.*, 2013). The typical lifespan of wolves is shorter than that of domesticated dogs and, although many factors are responsible for mortality in wolves and dogs, this evidence is not consistent with a significant benefit for raw food over proprietary food. Therefore, further work is required before any perceived advantages of a so-called 'ancestral diet' can be clarified.
- Can be carbohydrate/gluten/wheat free
  - Unlike wolves, domesticated dogs can readily digest carbohydrates; 10 of the 36 genomic differences between these species are involved in carbohydrate digestion (Axelsson *et al.*, 2013). Studies have shown that cats can also utilize carbohydrates, but to a lesser extent than dogs (Morris *et al.*, 1977). True dietary intolerances are rare and generally assumed to be related to the protein component rather than the carbohydrate component of the diet (August, 1985; Hodgkins, 1991; Harvey, 1993) (see Chapter 14).
- Improved stool volume
  - There may be a smaller stool volume in pets fed RMBDs due to the lower fibre content of the diet (Vester *et al.*, 2010; Freeman *et al.*, 2013).
- Reduced faecal odour
  - Raw diets may reduce flatulence. This is thought to be due to having typically less fermentable fibre (Ugarte *et al.*, 2004). However, as a result of having less ferment-able fibre, RMBDs might result in decreased short-chain fatty acid production. This may be detrimental to the pet because short-chain fatty acids are essential for large intestinal health (see Chapter 18).
- Can be fed at all life stages
  - Some commercial producers of RMBDs make different products for different life stages. Homemade BARF-type diets are advertised as 'all-life' products. This implies that the recipe is suitable for young, old, pregnant, lactating, healthy or sick individuals. However, this is not necessarily advisable, and any recipe should be formulated for the life stage of the pet, ideally by an appropriately qualified individual (see Chapter 1).

Disadvantages of feeding a raw meat-based diet

The risks associated with feeding RMBDs include:

- Risk of multidrug-resistant bacteria
  - There are associated risks to the pet, owners and extended families, as well as veterinary and hospital staff. The multidrug-resistant bacteria of particular concern include *Escherichia coli* (*E. coli*) and meticillin-resistant *Staphylococcus pseudintermedius* (MRSP) (Bos *et al.*, 2019; Morgan *et al.*, 2024b).

- Risk of pathogenic infection
  - Concerns regarding the risk of pathogenic infection from RMBDs have been frequently raised (Davies *et al.*, 2019). An online survey taking a closer look at pet owners' perceptions of feeding RMBDs and the incidence of infection has suggested that the risks appear to be low, although not negligible (Anturaniemi *et al.*, 2019).

Pathogenic infection

Although not common, cases of pets contracting *Salmonella* spp. and other pathogens has been reported (Caraway *et al.*, 1959; Stone *et al.*, 1993; Cantor *et al.*, 1997; Clark *et al.*, 2001; Joffe and Schlesinger, 2002) (Figure 6.2). Risks to owners arise not only from the handling of uncooked food, but also from handling the pet – contact with the pet's saliva, fur, urine and faeces are points of concern.

- Pathogens are shed by the pet during urination and defecation (Figure 6.3). During grooming, the pet may spread pathogens to their coat via their saliva. Pathogens may also be shed asymptomatically into the environment where the pet lives or has contact with, which might be a further source of spread.
- In one study 21–48% of home-prepared and commercially produced RMBDs tested were found to have pathogenic contamination (Weese *et al.*, 2005; Finley *et al.*, 2008).
- The freezing of pet foods does not guarantee food safety, as commonly thought, because it does not eliminate all pathogens that may be harmful. Freezing decreases *Campylobacter* colony counts, but will not completely eradicate it or other pathogens, most of which are unaffected by freezing (Finley *et al.*, 2008).
- High hydrostatic pressure processing or high pressure pasteurization is a process used by some commercial RMBD producers to reduce pathogen risk. However, it does not completely eradicate all pathogens and it is thought that it may lead to pathogenic resistance (van Bree *et al.*, 2018).
- Some proponents of RMBDs argue that the risk of pathogens from raw feeding is no greater than from any foods intended for human consumption. However, while there is undoubtedly a risk, it is arguably reduced because such food is usually cooked when consumed by humans. Furthermore, the risks associated with feeding raw food arise not only from the food but also from owner contact with the pet.
- Some proponents of raw feeding argue that contamination of pet food with pathogens is more common with conventional commercial foods, which are cooked. While this might be correct when examining the absolute number of pet food withdrawals, it should be noted that this is because such foods are much more commonly fed. Relatively speaking, many more come from raw food manufacturers.
- Based on available evidence, the risk of pathogenic infection should be considered when recommending a raw diet. Arguably, the potential risk to human health may be more of a concern than the risk to dogs and cats consuming the raw diet. The prevalence of such infections is unknown, as it is not frequently reported, or in some cases the cause may not be associated with the pet or its food. Therefore, owners who wish to feed a RMBD should be strongly advised to take adequate precautions to reduce this risk.

Potential concerns from specific ingredients

Although known to be rare, there are some potential risks associated with specific ingredients in a raw diet (Figure 6.4). It is important that owners wishing to feed a RMBD recognize these risks.

Pathogen	Risk
Salmonella spp.	Between 4% and 10% of chicken produced and sold in the United Kingdom (UK) for human consumption carries *Salmonella* spp. Amounts found on imported chicken are higher still (Food Standards Agency, 2003). Many studies have confirmed the transmission of *Salmonella* to pets in the contaminated meats that they are fed (Caraway *et al.*, 1959; Stone *et al.*, 1993; Cantor *et al.*, 1997; Clark *et al.*, 2001; Joffe and Schlesinger, 2002). Simple cleaning of food bowls at home with soap and water or in a dishwasher is not sufficient to eliminate this pathogen. Although uncommon, cases of zoonotic infection of *Salmonella* to pet owners has been linked with feeding a raw diet to the family pet (Minnesota Department of Health, 2018). Most pets that become infected with *Salmonella* become asymptomatic carriers, but studies have shown that they will still shed the bacteria in their saliva and faeces for 7 days after each infectious incident (Verma *et al.*, 2007)
Escherichia coli	This pathogen was found in 60% of raw diets tested – both homemade and commercially produced (Freeman and Michel, 2001; Strohmeyer *et al.*, 2006). Human deaths have been reported from handling raw dog food contaminated with *E. coli* (Davies *et al.*, 2019)
Clostridium spp.	Although the pathogenic nature of *Clostridium* spp. remains unclear, 20% of commercially produced raw diets were found to carry these bacteria (Weese *et al.*, 2005)
Campylobacter jejuni	This pathogen is present in 50–70% of all chicken sold for human consumption in the UK (Food Standards Agency, 2016). Acute polyradiculoneuritis in dogs (a neurological disorder) is thought to be triggered by pathogenic infection of *Campylobacter* deriving from contaminated food fed to pets (Martinez-Anton *et al.*, 2018)
Toxoplasma gondii	This pathogen is especially dangerous for pregnant women (as it causes fetal abnormalities) and for immunosuppressed individuals. Women are advised to avoid direct contact with their cat's faeces and litter tray (as this is where the spread of the pathogen is most likely) during pregnancy (Gov.uk, 2008). As the prevalence of *Toxoplasma* in cats is greater when fed a raw diet, this should be given further consideration if living with at-risk individuals (Smielewska-Los *et al.*, 2002; Dubey *et al.*, 2005; Lopes *et al.*, 2008)
Listeria spp.	This pathogen is widely found in meat products sold for human consumption (Food Standards Agency, 2019a). Raw meat-based pet food products have been withdrawn for containing dangerous levels of this pathogen (Food Standards Agency, 2019b). Infection with *Listeria* spp. in humans causes a range of clinical signs from 'flu-like' to fatal meningitis and abortion during pregnancy
Mycobacterium bovis	Found in uncooked commercially manufactured raw cat food; it can cause a fatal infection in many cats (O'Halloran *et al.*, 2019)

Figure 6.2: Reported pathogenic infections when feeding a raw meat-based diet and the associated risks. (continues)

Pathogen	Risk
Yersinia enterocolitica; *Mycobacterium tuberculosis*; *Francisella tularensis* (causes tularaemia); and *Echinococcus multilocularis*	All pose a health risk to all groups of people having contact with the pet

Figure 6.2: (continued) Reported pathogenic infections when feeding a raw meat-based diet and the associated risks.

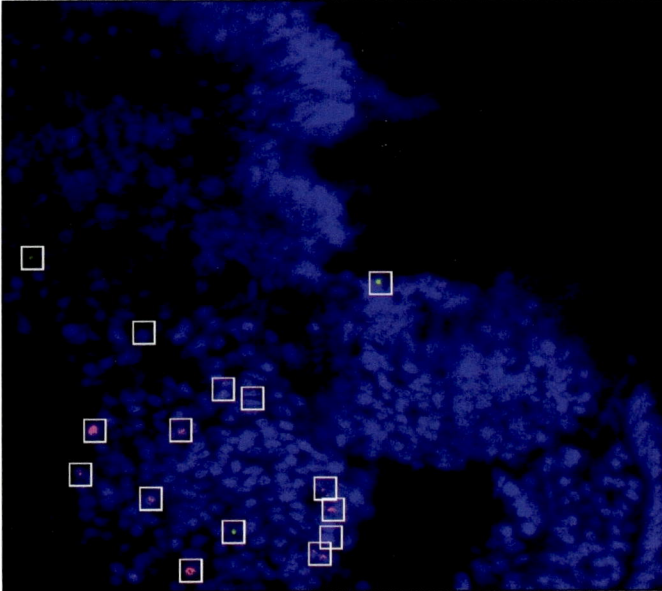

Figure 6.3: Fluorescent *in situ* hybridization (FISH) in a sample of small intestine from a dog with diarrhoea that had been fed a raw meat-based diet. The position of the bacteria are highlighted by the surrounding white boxes. A eubacterial probe shows green fluorescence and *Campylobacter* appears red.

Ingredient	Risk
Raw egg white	Contains avidin which binds to the B vitamin biotin making it unavailable. This may result in protein deficiency (Case *et al.*, 2000)
Some raw fish or shellfish	Contains thiaminase, which destroys the B vitamin thiamine causing protein deficiency (Case *et al.*, 2000)
Liver	Fed in large quantities can cause hypervitaminosis A due to the large amounts of vitamin A stored in liver tissue (Case *et al.*, 2000)
Gullet	Often contains the thyroid gland, which when fed can cause hyperthyroidism

Figure 6.4: Risks associated with specific ingredients of raw meat-based diets.

Excess or deficiency in the diet

When feeding a raw diet, especially if preparing it at home, it is very difficult for the owner to ensure that they are feeding a complete and balanced diet to their pet. Research to determine the nutritional adequacy of home-prepared foods, both cooked and uncooked, has found some concerning results:

- In one study where 95 different RMBDs were examined (Dillitzer *et al.*, 2011):
  - The majority of the diets (60%) were found to have a significant imbalance
  - Only 40% were balanced or had a minor imbalance.
- In two similar studies examining 94 commonly available recipes for home-prepared diets (both cooked and uncooked) for pets with medical conditions, all were found to be inadequate (Heinze *et al.*, 2012; Larsen *et al.*, 2012)
- In a further study of 200 different recipes for maintenance diets, 95% were deficient in at least one essential nutrient and 84% had multiple deficiencies (Stockman *et al.*, 2013).

Clinical signs associated with conditions that are caused by feeding an unbalanced diet can take a considerable period of time to appear. At this point the damage may be irreversible. Deficiencies include low calcium, which can occur when an all-meat, table-scrap or all organ-meat diet is fed. These diets, being very low in calcium, cause hypocalcaemia resulting in nutritional secondary hyperparathyroidism. This is a very painful condition leading to significant bone loss through demineralization and multiple pathological bone fractures (Bennett, 1976; Hintz and Schryver, 1987). Although there are no published studies on prevalence, the risk of obvious nutrient deficiencies in adult dogs and cats appear to be rare. However, such deficiencies are more frequently reported in growing animals and, as a result, caution should be exercised when feeding such diets to animals that have not yet reached skeletal maturity (see Chapter 10).

Owner compliance

As with any diet, compliance from owners will vary. Some diets can be inappropriate for pets as they include little or no carbohydrates, meaning that protein and/or fat concentrations have to be increased. Arguably, the greatest concern comes from home-prepared RMBDs. Not only are the recipes often unbalanced to begin with, but it can be difficult for owners to be fully compliant with the recipe (see Chapter 5).

Safety measures when feeding raw meat-based diets

Hygiene

A higher standard of hygiene is essential for the safe feeding of RMBDs compared with other diets due to the handling of raw ingredients.

- At purchase, the ingredient packaging should be inspected for damage or contamination. If apparent, the ingredient should not be purchased and should be discarded.
- Hand washing should be undertaken both before and after food preparation as well as after touching the pet.
- Preparation areas and surfaces should be cleaned with disinfectant immediately after the food has been prepared and, if possible, separate from human food preparation areas.

- Clean food bowls should be used for each meal.
- Bowls, floors and utensils should be disinfected immediately after feeding has finished (Figure 6.5).
- Bowls or plates for pet use should be kept separate from the ones used by the owners. Washing of bowls and plates alone is not enough to eliminate bacteria such as *Salmonella* (Weese and Rousseau, 2006).

Storage and feeding

Correct storage and feeding of RMBDs will reduce the cross-contamination risk.

- Uncooked foods should be defrosted in sealed containers (Figure 6.6) or in the pet's bowl, ensuring that it is covered.
- Thawed, uncooked foods should not be refrozen.
- The thaw juice should not be discarded as it contains nutrients and should be fed to the pet in the meal.
- Defrosted food must be stored in sealed containers and refrigerated (i.e. at the bottom of the refrigerator or, ideally, in a separate refrigerator – although this does not appear to be a contributing factor to the incidence of infection according to a recent study (Anturaniemi *et al.*, 2019)).

Due to its high moisture content and potential for pathogenic contamination, it is not advisable to feed RMBDs on an *ad libitum* basis. As with any food, an appropriate daily ration (based on the maintenance energy requirement of the dog or cat; see Chapter 2) should be fed in meals, with uneaten food being removed after 30 minutes, disposed of and never reoffered to the pet.

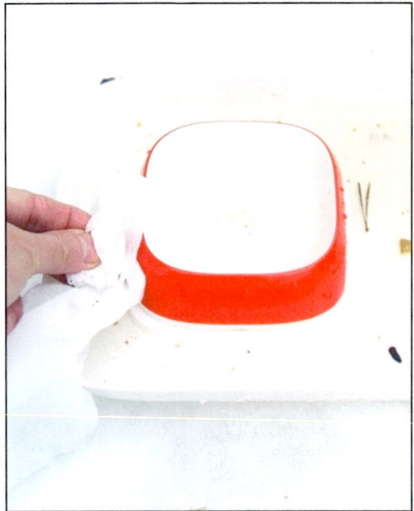

Figure 6.5: Food bowls should be cleaned and disinfected after every meal.
(Image used under the licence from Shutterstock.com: © victoras)

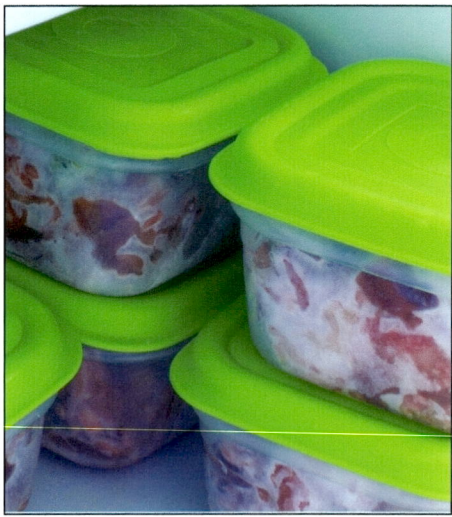

Figure 6.6: Raw food should be stored and defrosted in sealed containers.
(Image used under the licence from Shutterstock.com: © Swingout)

Handling

Care is needed when handling pets and areas that the pet has contact with, especially those used for elimination. Studies have shown that pets infected with pathogenic bacteria can shed them into the environment (Davies *et al.*, 2019). Therefore, the following precautions should be observed:

- Gloves should be worn or hands washed immediately after any handling or contact with urine or faeces
- Areas within the home where inappropriate elimination has occurred should be swiftly disinfected
- Elimination areas within the owner's garden should be fastidiously cleared or cleaned
- High general levels of environmental cleanliness and regular washing of bedding are also advisable, although further work is needed to ascertain whether washing is sufficient for pathogen removal
- Consideration should also be given to taking dogs to public areas, which may be difficult or impossible to clean (i.e. should these dogs be prevented from eliminating in public areas?).

Monitoring

It has been suggested that pets fed a RMBD could be tested regularly to screen for nutrient deficiencies. Tests should include biochemistry (including thyroxine concentrations), haematology and urinalysis. Adults may be tested every 6 to 12 months (Freeman *et al.*, 2013). However, it should be noted that unless the deficiencies are extreme, blood profiles may not identify them. Checking the diet history, or if the manufacturer of the diet is following the European Pet Food Industry Federation (FEDIAF) nutritional guidelines, will provide more information on whether there are likely to be deficiencies within the diet (Hajek V *et al.*, 2022).

Considerations for feeding raw diets

Healthy dogs and cats

Dietary requirements can vary greatly between the different life stages and, arguably, no one diet will provide optimal nutrition for all stages. It is strongly recommended to seek the advice of an appropriately qualified person (see Chapter 1) before feeding a RMBD to growing animals. This is likely the life stage where optimal nutrition is most critical.

Dogs and cats with various diseases

Patients with many different diseases have specific nutritional requirements, meaning that a RMBD may not be appropriate in such circumstances. For example:

- Chronic kidney disease (CKD)
  - CKD requires a diet with restricted phosphorus content and protein restriction should be considered at later stages (Polzin, 2019; see Chapter 19). This is extremely difficult to achieve with a RMBD since both the protein and phosphorus content can be very high.
- Obesity
  - Behavioural research indicates that dogs rarely regulate their food intake and will commonly overeat, especially when offered foods they find palatable (Roberts *et al.*, 2018). The greater fat and protein content of raw diets may mean such diets are overconsumed if fed *ad libitum*, leading to unwanted weight gain (see Chapter 15). While some cats will regulate their own intake, typically they consume more when fed higher protein diets (Beynen, 2015, 2018).

- Compromised immune system
  - Pets that may be immunocompromised include those with neoplasia and hyperadrenocorticism, as well as those being treated with corticosteroids.

Feeding raw meat-based diets in a hospital environment

As more dogs and cats are being fed RMBDs, it is important to consider the potential impact that this may have in a veterinary hospital (see Chapter 12). Many large hospitals and referral centres have adopted the following rules to reduce the risks to staff and other patients:

- No raw diets allowed into the hospital in order to:
  - Reduce risk to immunocompromised patients
  - Reduce cross-contamination risks to staff and other animals.
- Patients consuming a raw meat-based diet at home may need to be isolated:
  - Pets can shed pathogens asymptomatically for 7 days after eating contaminated meats.

Conclusion

The feeding of RMBDs has become increasingly popular in recent years. It is therefore vitally important that veterinary professionals first educate themselves on the available options, and then consider all the pros and cons when advising owners of the best diet to feed their pet. Decisions will often be made 'on balance' for the individual. Advice based on good evidence should be given each time and any recommendation must ensure that minimum nutritional requirements are met.

References and further reading

Allan F, Blake D, Miller Z and Church D (2022) Biliary protozoa in a dog with acute cholangiohepatitis fed a raw food diet. *Journal of Internal Veterinary Medicine* **36(6)**, 2177–2180

Anturaniemi J, Barrouin-Melo SM, Zaldivar-López S *et al.* (2019) Owners' perception of acquiring infections through raw pet food: a comprehensive internet-based survey. *Veterinary Record* **185**, 658

August JR (1985) Dietary hypersensitivity in dogs: cutaneous manifestations, diagnosis and management. *Compendium on Continuing Education for the Practicing Veterinarian* **7**, 469–477

Axelsson E, Ratnakumar A, Arendt ML *et al.* (2013) The genomic signature of dog domestication reveals adaptation to a starch-rich diet. *Nature* **495**, 360–364

Bennett D (1976) Nutrition and bone disease in the dog and cat. *Veterinary Record* **98**, 313–320

Beynen AC (2015) Dry foods for cats. *Creature Companion* **July**, 54–55

Beynen AC (2018) Cat food composition and caloric intake. *Dier-en-Arts Nr* **8/9**, 186–189

Billinghurst I (1993) *Give your dog a bone: the practical common-sense way to feed dogs for a long healthy life.* Bridge Printery, Alexandria NSW, Australia

Bojanić K, Acke E, Biggs PJ and Midwinter AC (2022) The prevalence of *Salmonella* spp. in working farm dogs and their home-kill raw meat diets in Manawatū, New Zealand. *New Zealand Veterinary Journal* **70(4)**, 233–237

Bos M, Broadfoot F, Healey K *et al.* (2019) *UK Veterinary Antimicrobial Resistance and Sales Surveillance.* [Available from: https:// www.gov.uk/ government/publications/ veterinary-antimicrobial-resistance-and-sales-surveillance-2018]

Candellone A, Badino P, Girolami F *et al.* (2023) Concomitant campylobacteriosis in a puppy and in its caregiver: a One Health perspective paridgm in human-pet relationship. *Veterinary Sciences* **10(4)**, 244

Cantor GH, Nelson Jr S, Vanek JA *et al.* (1997) *Salmonella* shedding in racing sled dogs. *Journal of Veterinary Diagnostic Investigation* **9(4)**, 447–448

Caraway CT, Scott AE, Roberts NC and Hauser GH (1959) Salmonellosis in sentry dogs. *Journal of the American Veterinary Medical Association* **135**, 599–602

Case LP, Carey DP, Hirakawa DA and Daristotle L (2000) *Canine and Feline Nutrition, 2nd edn.* Mosby Elsevier, Philadelphia

Clark C, Cunningham J, Ahmed R *et al.* (2001) Characterization of *Salmonella* associated with pig ear dog treats in Canada. *Journal of Clinical Microbiology* **39(11)**, 3962–3968

Cole SD, Healy I, Dietrich JM and Redding LE (2022) Evaluation of canine raw food products for the presence of extended-spectrum beta-lactamase and carbapenemase-producing bacteria of the order Enterobacterales. *American Journal of Veterinary Research* **83(9)**, doi: 10.2460/ajvr.21.12.0205

Commission Regulation (EU) 1334/2008 of the European Parliament and Council (2008) *On flavourings and certain food ingredients with flavouring properties for use in and on foods and amending Council Regulation (EEC) No. 1601/91, Regulations (EC) No. 2232/96 and (EC) No. 110/2008 and Directive 2000/13/EC.* [Available from: https://eur-lex.europa.eu/legal-content/ EN/ TXT/?qid=1585739671020&uri=CELEX:320 08R1334]

Davies RH, Lawes JR and Wales AD (2019) Raw diets for dogs and cats: a review with particular reference to microbiological hazards. *Journal of Small Animal Practice* **60**, 329–339

Dillitzer N, Becker N and Kienzle E (2011) Intake of minerals, trace elements and vitamins in bone and raw food rations in adult dogs. *British Journal of Nutrition* **106**, S53–S56

Dogs Naturally (2020) *Raw feeding dogs: 10 simple rules to get started.* [Available from: www. dogsnaturallymagazine. com/raw-feeding-primer]

Dubey JP, Hill DE, Jones JL *et al.* (2005) Prevalence of viable *Toxoplasma gondii* in beef, chicken and pork from retail meat stores in the United States: risk assessment to consumers. *Journal of Parasitology* **91**, 1082–1093

Finco DR, Brown SA, Crowell WA *et al.* (1992) Effects of dietary phosphorus and protein in dogs with chronic renal failure. *American Journal of Veterinary Research* **53(12)**, 2264–2271

Finley R, Reid-Smith R, Ribble C *et al.* (2008) The occurrence and antimicrobial susceptibility of Salmonellae isolated from commercially available canine raw food diets in three Canadian cities. *Zoonosis and Public Health* **55**, 462–469

Food Standards Agency (2003) *UK-wide Survey of Salmonella and Campylobacter contamination of fresh and frozen chicken on retail sale.* [Available from: www.food.gov.uk]

Food Standards Agency (2016) *A UK wide microbiological survey of Campylobacter contamination in fresh whole chilled chickens at retail sale.* [Available from: https://www.food.gov.

uk/sites/default/files/media/document/retail_survey_protocol_year3_0.pdf]

Food Standards Agency (2019a) *Listeria cases being investigated.* [Available from: https://www.food. gov.uk/news-alerts/ news/ listeria-cases-being-investigated]

Food Standards Agency (2019b) *Raw Treat Pet Food Ltd recalls frozen raw beef, chicken, lamb, and chicken and tripe pet food due to the presence of Listeria monocytogenes.* [Available from: https:// www.food.gov.uk/news-alerts/alert/ fsaprin-36-2019]

Freeman LM, Chandler ML, Hamper BA and Weeth LP (2013) Current knowledge about the risks and benefits of raw meat based diets for dogs and cats. *Journal of the American Veterinary Medical Association* **243(11)**, 1549–1558

Freeman LM and Michel KE (2001) Evaluation of raw food diets for dogs. *Journal of the American Veterinary Medical Association* **218**, 705–709 (Erratum published in *Journal of the American Veterinary Medical Association* **218**, 1582)

German AJ, Woods GRT, Holden SL *et al.* (2018) Dangerous trends in pet obesity. *Veterinary Record* **182**, 25

Gibson JF, Parker VJ, Howard JP *et al.* (2022) *Escherichia coli* pathotype contamination in raw canine diets. *American Journal of Veterinary Research* **83(6)**, doi: 10.2460/ajvr.21.10.0166

Gov.uk (2008) *Toxoplasmosis: diagnosis, epidemiology and prevention.* [Available from: www.gov.uk/guidance/ toxoplasmosis]

Groat EF, Williams NJ, Pinchbeck G, Warner B, Simpson A and Schmidt VM (2022) UK dogs eating raw meat diets have higher risk of *Salmonella* and antimicrobial-resistant *Escherichia coli* faecal carriage. *Journal of Small Animal Practice* **63(6)**, 435–441

Hajek V, Zablotski Y and Kölle P (2022) Computer-aided ration calculation (Diet Check Munich©) *versus* blood profile in raw fed privately owned dogs. *Journal of Animal Physiology and Animal Nutrition* **106(2)**, 345–354

Hamper BA, Kirk CA and Bartges JW (2016) Apparent nutrient digestibility of two raw diets in domestic kittens. *Journal of Feline Medicine and Surgery* **18(12)**, 991–996

Harvey RG (1993) Food allergy and dietary intolerance in dogs: a report of 25 cases. *Journal of Small Animal Practice* **34**, 175–179

Heinze CR, Gomez FC and Freeman LM (2012) Assessment of commercial diets and recipes for home-prepared diets recommended for dogs with cancer. *Journal of the American Veterinary Medical Association* **241**, 1453–1460

Hintz HF and Schryver HF (1987) Nutrition and bone development in dogs. *European Journal of Companion Animal Practice* **1**, 44–47

Hodgkins E (1991) Food allergy in cats: considerations, diagnosis and management. *Pet Vet* **24**, 8

Joffe DJ and Schlesinger DP (2002), Preliminary assessment of the risk of Salmonella infection in dogs fed raw chicken diets. Canadian Veterinary Journal **43(6)**, 441–442

Kendall PT and Holme DW (1982) Studies on digestibility of soya bean products, cereal, cereal and plant by-products in the diet of dogs. Journal of the Science of Food and Agriculture **33**, 813–820

Larsen JA, Parks EM, Heinze CR and Fascetti AJ (2012) Evaluation of recipes for home-prepared diets for dogs and cats with chronic kidney disease. Journal of the American Veterinary Medical Association **240**, 532–538

Lopes AP, Cardoso L and Rodrigues M (2008) Serological survey of Toxoplasma gondii infection in domestic cats from northeastern Portugal. Veterinary Parasitology **155**, 184–189

Martinez-Anton L, Marenda M, Firestone SM et al. (2018) Investigation of the role of Campylobacter infection in suspected acute polyradiculoneuritis in dogs. Journal of Veterinary Internal Medicine **32(1)**, 352–360

Marx FR, Machado GS, Pezzali JG et al. (2016) Raw beef bones as chewing items to reduce dental calculus in Beagle dogs. Australian Veterinary Journal **94(1–2)**, 18–23

Minnesota Department of Health (2018) Salmonella cases linked to raw meat dog food. [Available from: www.health.state.mn.us/news/pressrel/2018/salmonella020918]

Morgan G, Pinchbeck G, Haldenby S, Schmidt V and Williams N (2024a) Raw meat diets are a major risk factor for carriage of third-generation cephalosporin-resistant and multidrug-resistant E.coli by dogs in the UK. Frontiers in Microbiology **15**, 1460143

Morgan G, Pinchbeck G, Taymaz E et al. (2024b) An investigation of the presence and antimicrobial susceptibility of Enterobacteriaceae in raw and cooked kibble diets for dogs in the United Kingdom. Frontiers in Microbiology doi: 10.3389/fmicb.2023.1301841

Morris GJ, Trudell J and Pencovic T (1977) Carbohydrate digestion by the domestic cat (Felis catus). British Journal of Nutrition **37(3)**, 365–373

O'Halloran C, Ioannidi O, Reed N et al. (2019) Tuberculosis due to Mycobacterium bovis in pet cats associated with feeding a commercial raw diet. Journal of Feline Medicine and Surgery **21(8)**, 667–681

Polzin D (2019) International Renal Interest Society–Diets for Cats with Chronic Kidney Disease (CKD). [Available from: http://www.iris-kidney.com/education/protein_restriction_feline_ckd.html]

Purina (2017) What are Fillers in Dog Food? [Available from: www.justrightpetfood.com/blog/dog-food-fillers]

Ribeiro-Almeida M, Mourão, Magalhães M et al. (2024) Raw meat-based diet for pets: a neglected source of human exposure to Salmonella and pathogenic Escherichia coli clones carrying mcr, Portugal, September 2019 to January 2020. Euro Surveillance **29(18)**, doi: 10.2807/1560-7917.ES.2024.29.18.2300561

Roberts MT, Bermingham EN, Cave NJ et al. (2018) Macronutrient intake of dogs, self-selecting diets varying in composition offered ad libitum. Journal of Animal Physiology and Animal Nutrition **102(2)**, 568–575

Ross LA, Finco DR and Crowell WA (1982) Effect of phosphorus restriction on the kidneys of cats with reduced renal mass. American Journal of Veterinary Research **43(6)**, 1023–1026

Smielewska-Loś E, Rypuła K and Pacoń J (2002) The influence of feeding and maintenance system on the occurrence of Toxoplasma gondii infections in dogs. Polish Journal of Veterinary Sciences **5**, 231–234

Stockman J, Fascetti AJ, Kass PH et al. (2013) Evaluation of recipes of home-prepared maintenance diets for dogs. Journal of the American Veterinary Medical Association **242**, 1500–1505

Stone GG, Chengappa MM, Oberst RD et al. (1993) Application of polymerase chain reaction for the correlation of Salmonella serovars recovered from Greyhound faeces with their diet. Journal of Veterinary Diagnostic Investigation **5(3)**, 378–385

Strohmeyer RA, Morley PS, Hyatt DR et al. (2006) Evaluation of bacterial and protozoal contamination of commercially available raw meat diets for dogs. Journal of the American Veterinary Medical Association **228**, 537–542

Tuska-Szalay B, Papdeák V, Vizi Z, Takács N and Hornok S (2024) Parasitological and molecular investigation of consequences of raw meat feeding (BARF) in dogs and cats: implications for other pets living nearby. Parasitology research **123(2)**, 114

Ugarte C, Guilford WG, Markwell P and Lupton E (2004) Carbohydrate malabsorption is a feature of feline inflammatory bowel disease but does not increase clinical gastrointestinal signs. Journal of Nutrition **8**, 2068S

van Bree FPJ, Bokken GCAM, Mineur R et al. (2018) Zoonotic bacterial and parasites found in raw meat-based diets for cats and dogs. Veterinary Record **182(2)**, 50

Verma AK, Sinha DK and Singh BR (2007) Salmonellosis in apparently healthy dogs. Journal of Veterinary Public Health **5(1)**, 37–39

Vester BM, Burke SL, Liu KJ et al. (2010) Influence of feeding raw or extruded feline diets on nutrient digestibility and nitrogen metabolism of African wildcats (Felis lybica). Zoo Biology **29**, 676–686

Weese JS and Rousseau J (2006) Survival of Salmonella Copenhagen in food bowls following contamination with experimentally inoculated raw meat: effects of time, cleaning and disinfection. The Canadian Veterinary Journal **47(9)**, 887–889

Weese JS, Rousseau J and Arroyo L (2005)
Bacteriological evaluation of commercial canine
and feline raw diets. *Canadian Veterinary Journal*
46, 513–516

Yukawa S, Uchida I, Takemitsu *et al.* (2022)
Anti-microbial resistance of *Salmonella* isolates
from raw meat-based dog food in Japan.
Veterinary Medicine and Science **8(3)**, 982–989

Online extras

This chapter includes:

- **A client information leaflet that is available to download and print from the BSAVA Library**

Access via QR code or: bsavalibrary.com/nutrition_6

Plant-based diets

7

Plant-based diets, for dogs at least, appear to offer some possible practical and partial solutions to the problems associated with the environmental impact of producing pet foods. However, this is not without drawbacks and nutritional challenges, particularly for cats. Although such diets may feature more heavily in the way owners feed their pets in the future, further work is required before they can be widely recommended. Not uncommonly, vegetarian or vegan pet food is chosen because that is the food type consumed by the owner, which extends from their belief system (The Vegan Society, 2022); religious or cultural considerations may also inform diet choice. As a result, products derived from, associated with, or tested on animals are avoided (e.g. meat, dairy, eggs, honey).

Plant-based diets comprise cooked and some uncooked ingredients including:

- **Vegetarian diets**
  - Green and/or yellow vegetables
  - Root vegetables
  - Legumes
  - Cereals
  - Nuts
  - Oils
  - Seeds
  - Fruits
  - Dairy products
  - Eggs
  - No meat-based products including products derived from animals such as gelatine.

- **Vegan diets**
  - As above with the exclusion of dairy products and eggs
  - No meat-based products including products derived from animals such as honey or gelatine.

In recent years, the importance of maintaining human health by eating a diet high in fruits and vegetables has been emphasized (e.g. the National Health Service (NHS) 5-a-day campaign; NHS England, 2022). Some studies have also suggested that vegan diets may be a healthy option for pets (Knight *et al.*, 2022); however, it should be noted that the studies undertaken to date have been short-term, observational and have relied on potentially biased owner self-reporting via surveys. Further, other studies re-analysing the same data have disputed these findings (Barrett-Jolley and German, 2024; German and Barrett-Jolley 2024). The results, therefore, should be interpreted cautiously, not least because the associations identified do not prove causality. Vegan diets differ in nutrient formulation from other commercially manufactured options (e.g. dry food); not only will the ingredient source be different, but additional mineral and amino acid supplements may be required.

Nonetheless, these studies do not suggest that provision of a vegetarian or vegan diet leads to obvious poorer health with short-term feeding. That said, many concerns have been raised about the nutritional adequacy of vegetarian and vegan diets, particularly for cats.

Sustainability and ethical concerns

Meat production places a significant toll on the environment. This occurs with the use of pesticides, fertilizers and pharmaceuticals, as well as loss of natural land through deforestation to make way for livestock farmland and agricultural crop production (Figure 7.1). Deforestation, in turn, causes loss of wildlife due to the reduction of natural habitat and loss of biodiversity of both plants and animals in the area (Petrović *et al.*, 2015). The carbon footprint of meat production (and pet food production) is thought to be further contributing to global warming (Röös *et al.*, 2013).

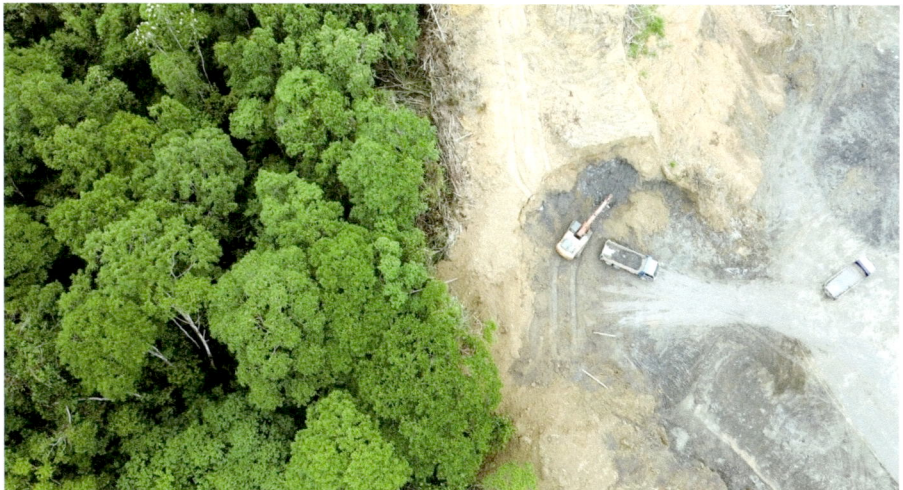

Figure 7.1: Deforestation contributes to the environmental impact of meat production for pet food. (Image used under the licence from Shutterstock.com © Rich Carey)

Due to the environmental impact, meat production at its current level may not be sustainable in the future. There is grave concern that, should meat consumption by both humans and pets continue as it is currently, meat shortages will be experienced within the next 50 years (Henchion *et al.*, 2017). In addition, as pets receive meats that are fit for human consumption, the competition for meat sources further increases. This has led many to consider alternative diets and ways of feeding their pets. Meat derivatives (by-products, i.e. the parts of an animal that humans choose not to eat) are often disposed of despite being nutritious. Therefore, to better sustain human meat consumption, increased meat derivative use would be an environmentally beneficial way to utilize these ingredients.

Producing meat products inevitably means that animals are slaughtered. Many concerns arise from the conditions animals are kept in prior to slaughter. In the United Kingdom (UK), methods of animal slaughter are regulated and overseen by the Food Standards Agency (FSA). Throughout the process, the FSA regularly inspects animals intended for slaughter for meat to ensure the welfare of the livestock.

Advantages of feeding a plant-based diet

- A suitable diet avoiding the need to feed animal-based products to dogs
  - The evidence suggests that it may be possible to meet all nutrient requirements for dogs using an appropriately formulated diet based solely on plant-based ingredients (Dodd *et al.*, 2018). Even extremely active sled dogs appear to be sustained well on short-term feeding of plant-based diets (Brown *et al.*, 2009). However, further work is recommended to confirm health and safety, including use for long-term feeding.
- A suitable diet avoiding the need to feed animal-based products to cats
  - Cats, as a carnivorous species, have specific requirements for nutrients that can only be found in meat-based ingredients. However, recently, non-animal sources for some of these nutrients have been suggested. For example, seaweed is rich in taurine and could be used as an alternative to taurine from an animal source. Other essential nutrients, such as vitamin A and arachidonic acid, can be manufactured synthetically. The bioavailability of these ingredients to cats has not been demonstrated in feeding trials, however, meaning that the safety of such diets cannot be assured. In addition, formulation is often problematic meaning that these diets frequently do not meet either the European Pet Food Industry Federation (FEDIAF) or the Association of American Feed Control Officials (AAFCO) recommendations for cats, especially during the growth phase.
- Reduced environmental impact
  - When compared with using meat-based ingredients, producing a pet food only from plant-based ingredients might reduce its environmental impact. However, these ingredients still have an impact and are not without concerns.
- More sustainable and environmentally friendly
  - Due to increasing competition and the unsustainable nature of meat production, together with its increasing environmental impact, greater use of plant-based or other ingredients in pet foods could be a more sustainable and environmentally friendly option. Many environmentalists suggest that urgent action is needed.

> **Note**
> Based on the current available evidence, it is not clear whether plant-based diets are either suitable or safe for cats, therefore, **sole feeding of such foods is not recommended**.

Disadvantages of feeding a plant-based diet

- Nutritional adequacy of plant-based diets
  - Concerns about the nutritional adequacy of plant-based diets are greatest for those diets formulated at home, where the risk of nutritional deficiency is significant (Larsen *et al.*, 2012). If such diets are to be considered, it is strongly recommended that guidance be sought from an individual with a suitable qualification (see Chapter 1). Research has shown that many of the commercially produced plant-based diets for cats and dogs may also be nutritionally inadequate (Zafalon *et al.*, 2020). As more manufacturers start producing this type of diet, further work to ensure nutritional adequacy is likely to be undertaken.

Some commonly used dietetic foods for dogs and cats are already based predominantly on plant-based ingredients (e.g. hydrolysed diets based on soya protein) and these have been used safely for many years. Therefore, nutritional adequacy (especially for dogs) may well be fully achievable.

- Urinary crystal and urolith formulation
  - Since plant-based proteins may result in a more alkaline urine than meat-based proteins, adaptations to the diet formulation might be needed to prevent urolith struvite formation. It would be prudent, therefore, to monitor the urinary health of individuals on a plant-based diet, particularly if they are prone to urolith formation (see Chapter 20).
- Environmental impact – soya bean production
  - Soya bean is already widely used globally as a protein source for both humans and animals and may be considered to be a more environmentally friendly option to proteins derived from meat production; however, many factors should be considered when determining how environmentally friendly an ingredient is. Most of the soya bean produced (77%) is fed to animals, with lesser amounts being consumed by humans (19%) or used in industry (4%) and only 0.5% is used to feed pets. Soya bean production requires considerable land (Figure 7.2) and, therefore, can be associated with deforestation, loss of wildlife and loss of biodiversity of plants and animal species, as well as use of pesticides and fertilizers (Figure 7.3) that can pollute the environment (Ritchie and Roser, 2021). Thus, although plant-based ingredients, such as soya bean may appear to be a more sustainable choice, they can still pose a significant environmental impact.

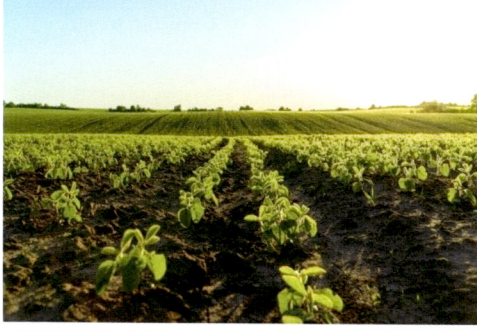

Figure 7.2: Soya bean production requires a large amount of land.
(Image used under the licence from Shutterstock.com © Jenya Smyk)

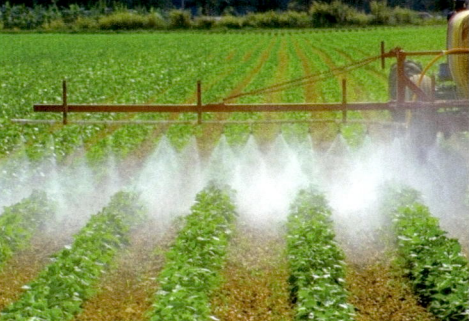

Figure 7.3: Soya bean field being sprayed with pesticides and fertilizers.
(Image used under the licence from Shutterstock.com © Dennis MacDonald)

Safety measures when feeding plant-based diets

Patients being fed plant-based diets should be regularly monitored. This may involve regular urine and blood testing (Figure 7.4ab). However, routine biochemistry and haematology are not sufficient to determine nutrient deficiencies; specific nutrient testing is required, which may be very costly. To get help with assessing the safety and suitability of a plant-based diet, or with how to ensure the diet is complete and balanced, assistance should be sought from an individual with a suitable qualification (see Chapter 1).

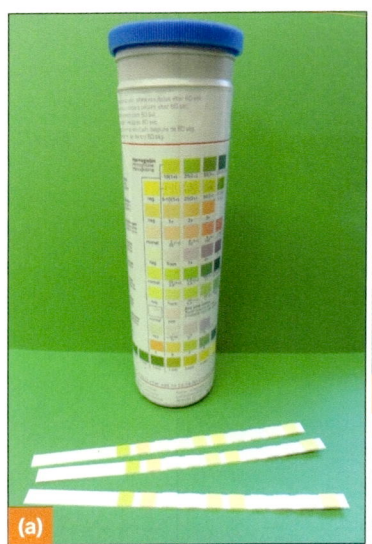

(a)

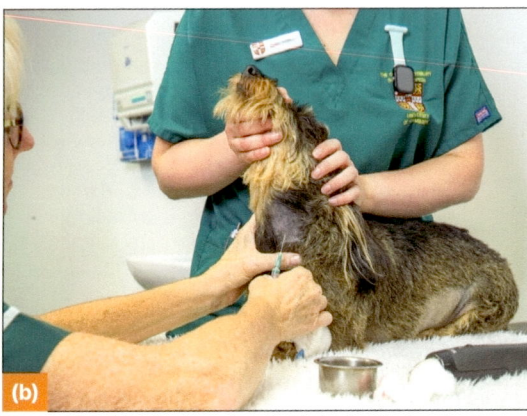

(b)

Figure 7.4: Monitoring of patients being fed a plant-based diet should be undertaken regularly and may include (a) urine testing and (b) blood testing.
(a, Reproduced from the *BSAVA Manual of Canine and Feline Clinical Pathology*; b, Reproduced from the BSAVA *Guide to Procedures in Small Animal Practice*)

Considerations for feeding plant-based diets

Healthy dogs

Nutritional inadequacy remains the biggest concern with the use of plant-based diets for both dogs and cats. This is particularly the case for growing animals where optimal nutrition is critical; for example, deficiencies in essential nutrients such as calcium can have catastrophic skeletal effects (Zafalon *et al.*, 2020). Thus, the use of vegetarian or vegan diets is not currently recommended for this age group. The current evidence suggests that it may be possible to use vegetarian and vegan diets safely in healthy adult dogs. However, given that some nutritional deficiencies take a considerable amount of time to develop, monitoring is key. Deficiencies may not manifest as overt clinical signs for months or even years, by which point the effects may be irreversible.

Healthy cats

Nutritional inadequacy

Cats are an obligate carnivore species (Bradshaw *et al.*, 1996). They have a greater requirement for proteins than dogs, as well as for nutrients that can only be found in animal-based products. Such nutrients include:

- Arginine
- Taurine
- Methionine
- Cystine
- Arachidonic acid
- Niacin
- Vitamin D
- Preformed retinol – vitamin A (as cats are unable to convert beta-carotene to vitamin A; Green *et al.*, 2012).

All these nutrients are naturally available in ingredients from animal sources, although there are natural plant-based sources for some of them. However, as mentioned above, the bioavailability of such nutrients is questionable (Michel, 2006). Whilst not perfect, appropriately conducted feeding trials (e.g. based on AAFCO protocols) are the only way of ensuring food safety, but, to the author's knowledge, none of the available vegetarian or vegan cat foods have yet been subject to such feeding trials (see Chapter 3).

Ethical considerations

Some people have argued that feeding a plant-based diet to cats might be unethical given that it is at odds with their natural physiology and behaviour (Bennett, 2021). The predatory instincts of cats have remained throughout their domestication, not least because of their use for pest control. As a result, cats differ very little genetically from their wild ancestor, the African Wildcat (Figure 7.5). The impact of feeding a plant-based diet on the behaviour of cats is not known, although there is some evidence that provision of a diet with a high meat content reduces predation of wildlife by domestic cats (Cecchetti *et al.*, 2021).

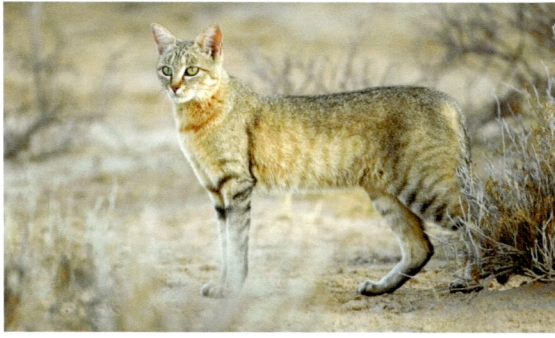

Figure 7.5: Domesticated cats genetically differ very little from their wild ancestor, the African Wildcat (*Felis silvestris lybica*).
(Image used under the licence from Shutterstock.com © EcoPrint)

Poor palatability

As cats did not evolve to consume plant-based foods, with some ingredient exceptions (e.g. pumpkin, courgette), plant-based diets may be unpalatable when fed in their natural state. Thus, palatability of a diet based on plant-based ingredients might be poor. That said, when it comes to diets that are commercially manufactured, this can be improved by the addition of palatants.

Dogs and cats with various diseases

Any pet with a disease is significantly impacted by the nutrition they receive. Healing and recovery are greatly reduced when a nutritional deficiency is present. Thus, it is even more important that patients with any illness or disease are provided with a safe, suitable, complete and balanced diet. In some circumstances, plant-based ingredients can be advantageous:

- **Liver disease:**
  - In the case of liver disease associated with hepatic encephalopathy in dogs, plant-based (or dairy-based) protein sources such as soya bean are preferable because they reduce the volume of ammonia produced during digestion, which must be eliminated by the liver. Plant-based proteins produce less ammonia than meat-based proteins, and so are often chosen in these instances (Proot *et al.*, 2009) (see Chapter 21).
- **Adverse reactions to food:**
  - Should an adverse reaction to food develop towards an animal protein source, the use of a plant-based protein source such as rice or soya bean could be an excellent option to eliminate feeding the ingredient that caused the clinical signs of the adverse reaction (see Chapter 14).
- **Obesity:**
  - Management of obesity requires calorie restriction and nutrient adaptations, alongside other environmental changes (see Chapter 15). As a result, any extra foods given by the pet owner as treats can slow or prevent weight loss. Green watery vegetables, which are readily accepted by most dogs, can make a good option to use as treats or to add bulk to the food allocation, helping the dog to feel full and the pet owner to manage food-seeking behaviours. Cats may also accept vegetables as treats, which can be advantageous during controlled weight reduction. In addition, green watery vegetables increase water intake which is often desirable. Additional foods should not make up more than 10% of the daily caloric intake
  - It should be noted that little nutritional value is derived from using vegetables in this way and all nutrients are obtained from the dietetic food that the pet should be consuming for safe weight loss. The vegetables are used solely for management of food-seeking behaviours, increasing feelings of satiety with each meal and/or increasing water intake. However, some vegetables can add to or complicate the nutritional balance (e.g. potassium in sweet potatoes, protein in mushrooms) and this should be taken into consideration.

Conclusion

Plant-based diets have the potential to offer some solutions to the problems associated with the environmental impact of producing pet foods. However, this is not without drawbacks and nutritional challenges. Further work is therefore needed before these diets can be widely recommended.

References and further reading

Barrett-Jolley R and German AJ (2024) Variables associated with owner perceptions of the health of their dog: further analysis of data from a large international survey *PLoS One* **19(5)**, e0280173

Bennett LK (2021) The legal, ethical and welfare implications of feeding vegan diets to dogs and cats. *The Veterinary Nurse* **12**, 108–114

Bexfield N and Riggs L (2024) *BSAVA Guide to Procedures in Small Animal Practice, 3rd edn.* BSAVA Publications, Gloucester

Bradshaw JWS, Goodwin D, Legrand-Defrétin V and Nott HMR (1996) Food selection by the domestic cat, an obligate carnivore. *Comparative Biochemistry and Physiology. Part A, Physiology* **114**, 205–209

Brown WY, Vanselow BA, Redman AJ and Pluske JR (2009) An experimental meat-free diet maintained haematological characteristics in sprint-racing sled dogs. *The British Journal of Nutrition* **102**, 1318–1323

Cecchetti M, Crowley, S L, Goodwin CED and McDonald RA (2021) Provision of high meat content food and object play reduce predation of wild animals by domestic cats (*Felis catus*). *Current Biology* **31(5)** 1107–1111

Dodd SAS, Adolphe JL and Verbrugghe A (2018) Plant-based diets for dogs. *Journal of the American Veterinary Medical Association* **253**, 1425–1432

German AJ and Barrett-Jolley R (2024) So, are vegan foods really healthier for dogs? *BSAVA Companion* **24(9)**, 20–24

Green AS, Tang G, Lango J, Klasing KC and Fascetti AJ (2012) Domestic cats convert [2H8]-β-carotene to [2H4]-retinol following a single oral dose. *Journal of Animal Physiology and Animal Nutrition (Berl)* **96**, 681–692

Henchion M, Hayes M, Mullen AM, Fenelon M and Tiwari B (2017) Future protein supply and demand: Strategies and factors influencing a sustainable equilibrium. *Foods* **6**, 1–21

Knight A, Huang E, Rai N and Brown H (2022) Vegan *versus* meat-based dog food: Guardian-reported indicators of health. *PLoS One* **17**

Larsen JA, Parks EM, Heinze CR and Fascetti AJ (2012) Evaluation of recipes for home-prepared diets for dogs and cats with chronic kidney disease. *Journal of the American Veterinary Medical Association* **240**, 532–538

Michel KE (2006) Unconventional diets for dogs and cats. *Veterinary Clinics of North America: Small Animal Practice* **36**, 1269–1281

NHS England (2022) *5-a-day campaign*. [Available from: https://www.nhs.uk/live-well/eat-well/5-a-day/]

Petrović Z, Djordjević V, Milicević D, Nastasijević I and Parunović N (2015) Meat production and consumption. Environmental consequences. *Procedia Food Science* **5**, 235–238

Proot S, Biourge V, Teske E and Rothuizen J (2009) Soy protein isolate *versus* meat-based low-protein diet for dogs with congenital portosystemic shunts. *Journal of Veterinary Internal Medicine* **23**, 794–800

Ritchie and Roser (2021) *Soy. Our World in Data.* [Available from: https://ourworldindata.org/soy]

Röös E, Sundberg C, Tidåker P, Strid I and Hansson PA (2013) Can carbon footprint serve as an indicator of the environmental impact of meat production? *Ecological Indicators* **24**, 573–581

The Vegan Society (2022) *Vegan animal care report* [Available from: https://www.vegansociety.com/resources/downloads]

Villiers E and Ristić J (2016) *BSAVA Manual of Canine and Feline Clinical Pathology, 3rd edn.* BSAVA Publications, Gloucester

Zafalon RVA, Risolia LW, Vendramini THA *et al.* (2020) Nutritional inadequacies in commercial vegan foods for dogs and cats. *PLoS One* **15**, 1–18

Online extras

This chapter includes:

- **A client information leaflet that is available to download and print from the BSAVA Library**

Access via QR code or: bsavalibrary.com/nutrition_7

Alternative protein-based diets

8

Alternative protein-based diets are typically commercially manufactured diets that offer a potentially more sustainable choice for owners concerned about the environmental impact of using animal proteins in pet food. These diets may become a common choice in the future. Alternative protein sources may provide the whole or partial protein source within the diet and are often plant-based or insect-based.

- **Plant-based protein sources**
  - Soya bean (Figure 8.1a)
  - Rice
  - Pea
  - Cereals
  - Algae (Figure 8.1b)
  - Fungi
  - Seitan (made from wheat gluten; Figure 8.1c)
  - Fruit by-products.

- **Insect-based protein sources**
  - Black soldier fly larvae (BSFL) (*Hemetia ilucens*; Figure 8.2a)
  - House crickets (*Acheta domesticus*; Figure 8.2b)
  - Yellow mealworms (*Tenebrio molitor*; Figure 8.2c)
  - Mulberry silkworms (*Bombyx mori*; Figure 8.2d).

- **Animal-based alternative protein sources**
  - Meat by-products (e.g. feathers)
  - Cultured meats
  - Invasive species (e.g. Asian carp).

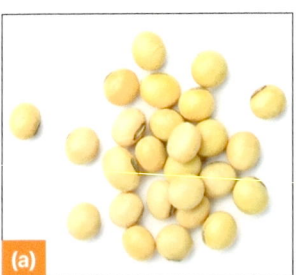 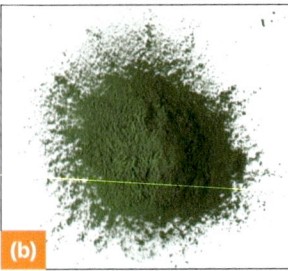 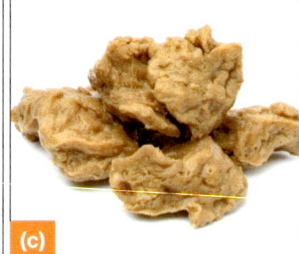

Figure 8.1: Examples of plant-based proteins used in pet food: (a) soya bean, (b) algae (spirulina) and (c) seitan.
(Images used under the licence from Shutterstock.com: (a) © Photoongraphy, (b) © xpixel and (c) © Picturepartners)

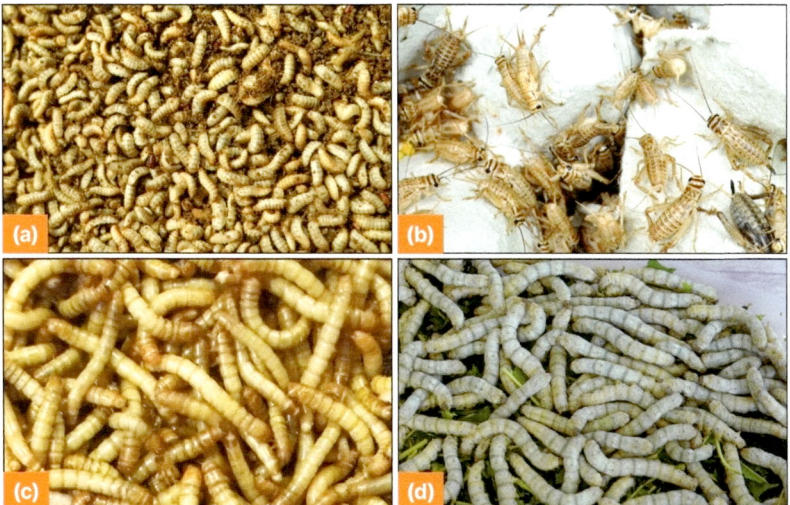

Figure 8.2: Examples of insect-based proteins used in pet food: (a) black soldier fly larvae, (b) house crickets, (c) yellow mealworms and (d) silkworms.
(Images used under the licence from Shutterstock.com: (a) © Hanif Ans, (b) © marima, (c) © bymaharrina and (d) © La Huertina De Toni)

There are many claims regarding alternative proteins that may make owners choose these diets above others.

As more is understood about the impact humans are having on the planet, there is arguably a need to decrease the effect of food production. A frequent concern is the significant carbon footprint created by commercial meat production (Alexander *et al.*, 2020) meaning that more environmentally friendly, sustainable options need to be available. Alternative sources of protein which can be farmed in vertical structures (e.g. BSFL and crickets), reduce the land mass required and the need for deforestation, as well as reduce pollution of water sources given that there is no longer a need for pesticides, fertilizers or antimicrobial drugs. As the environmental impact of using alternative protein sources is less in the long-term, these sources will become a more sustainable way to feed pets. If changes are not made to the way pets are fed, it is estimated that within the next 50 years there will be meat shortages that will affect both pets and humans.

There is also the perception that foods based on alternative proteins are 'less likely' to cause a hypersensitivity reaction. Many pet owners may choose an alternative protein diet because they think it might reduce the risk of digestive disturbances or pruritus. However, despite its widespread use in pet food marketing, there is no legal definition of the term 'hypoallergenic' and, to the author's knowledge, there is no evidence that such proteins are truly 'hypoallergenic'. Further, adverse reactions to food cannot be prevented by feeding alternative proteins. That said, such diets would be a logical choice when managing cats and dogs already diagnosed with adverse reactions to food because the protein is likely to be novel (see Chapters 4 and 14).

Owners increasingly want to know what their pet is consuming and may want their animal's diet to align with their own belief system; for example, some pet owners who consume vegan or vegetarian diets themselves, might prefer to avoid feeding their pet a diet containing animal products (see Chapter 7).

Advantages of feeding an alternative protein-based diet

- Wider selection of protein sources
  - Some alternative protein sources (e.g. soya bean, rice, peas, cereals) have been used in pet foods for many years. More recent research has examined the use of some plant-based (e.g. algae; McCusker *et al.*, 2014) and insect-based (e.g. BSFL) protein sources. The Association of American Feed Control Officials (AAFCO) and the European Pet Food Industry Federation (FEDIAF) have approved the use of BSFL, house crickets and yellow mealworms in pet foods for dogs and cats. With increasing consumer and environmental pressures, the approval of other protein sources is bound to follow (Areerat *et al.*, 2021); this will provide the pet food industry with a much wider choice of protein sources. In addition, the use of invasive species (such as Asian carp) as a protein source could also be considered.
- Novel protein sources
  - As some alternative protein sources are new to the market, it is unlikely that pets will have encountered them before. If this is the case, these ingredients could be utilized as a novel protein source (e.g. for the management of an adverse reaction to food; see Chapter 14), although further studies are required. In addition, further work is needed to determine the risks of cross-reactive allergies that have been identified (e.g. between mealworms and dust mites; Bajuk *et al.*, 2021).
- Highly digestible
  - Soya bean (Stein *et al.*, 2008) and insect proteins (McCusker *et al.*, 2014) are highly digestible ingredients for both dogs and cats. Foods based on BSFL are also highly digestible and, although further testing is required, they appear to be safe to feed cats and dogs (Freel *et al.*, 2021).
- Improved animal welfare
  - There are many concerns surrounding the welfare of livestock used in meat production for pet foods; however, with the use of alternative protein sources (e.g. insect-based protein), welfare is considered to be better. In addition, the insect species used typically live in colonies in tight dark spaces making them good candidates for mass commercial production (Figure 8.3).
- Reduced antimicrobial use
  - Antimicrobial use in commercial meat production is thought to be contributing to and increasing antimicrobial resistance in both pets and humans (Kasimanickam *et al.*, 2021). Given that such drugs are not required for the production of most alternative protein sources, these options are a logical way to reduce the overall level of antimicrobial drugs entering the human food chain.
- Low-grade/waste food products can be turned into high-quality proteins
  - BSFL and other insects can consume vegetable and fruit by-products that would otherwise be discarded (Spranghers *et al.*, 2017) (Figure 8.4). Turning waste products into high-quality proteins to be used in pet foods can be environmentally beneficial and could reduce the quantity of waste products from the food-producing industry.
- Fast to produce
  - Raising meat from traditional sources usually takes several months, depending on the species. Alternative protein sources such as BSFL can be produced very quickly (i.e. in a number of days; Meneguz *et al.*, 2018). Thus, these sources of protein could be made readily available to meet the increasing demands of the pet food industry.
- Organic
  - Insects used for the production of protein can be fed vegetation and, if this comes from organic sources, the insect-based proteins could also be considered organic.

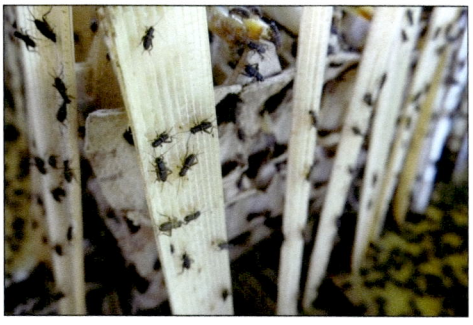

Figure 8.3: Crickets are farmed in tight colonies making them a more sustainable mass production source of protein.
(Image used under the licence from Shutterstock.com: © Ihlasul1411)

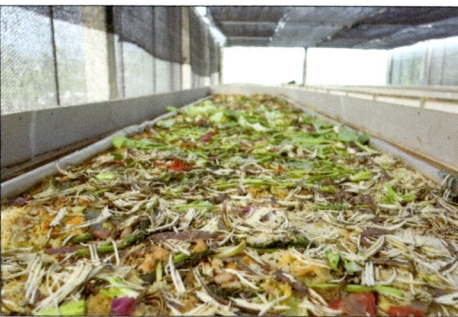

Figure 8.4: Black soldier fly larvae can be used to consume vegetable and fruit by-products. This is a sustainable and environmentally friendly method of biodegradable decomposition of waste materials.
(Image used under the licence from Shutterstock.com: © CardIrin)

Disadvantages of feeding an alternative protein-based diet

■ New concept
  • Since many of the alternative protein sources used in pet foods (e.g. insect-based products) are relatively new, little is known about the long-term impact of these diets. Further work is needed to confirm whether these diets are safe for pets at all stages of life, as well as for those with disease (where appropriate). However, other alternative protein sources (e.g. soya bean) are well established in canine and feline diets, including use in dietetic food (e.g. management of some types of liver disease (Norton *et al.*, 2016) and management of adverse reactions to food).
■ Availability
  • Currently, few diets use alternative protein sources, but this is likely to increase in the future as innovation and research progresses.
■ Environmental impact
  • Although insect-based proteins offer some meaningful environmental benefits, other protein sources such as soya bean, arguably have a negative environmental impact (Ritchie and Roser, 2021; see also Chapter 7).
■ Risk of dilated cardiomyopathy (DCM) in dogs
  • Recent work has highlighted an association between canine DCM (see Chapter 4) and the feeding of diets that contain protein from legumes such as peas and lentils. The mechanism for this remains unknown and, until further information is available, caution should be advised with feeding of these diets.

- Acceptance
  - In some cultures (e.g. Mexican), consuming insects is common (Ramos-Elorduv, 1997), but this is not the case elsewhere (e.g. Europe). Owners may be reluctant to feed insect protein to their pet, or to consume insects themselves, no matter what the nutritional value. Therefore, it might take time before some alternative proteins are accepted into the mainstream.

Safety measures when feeding alternative protein-based diets

As for any diet, those containing alternative proteins must fulfil all the nutritional requirements of the pet (see Chapter 1). Since these diets are most likely to be commercially produced, they must also satisfy all safety regulations that any other commercially manufactured product is required to meet (see Chapter 3). Biosecurity aspects of production also need to be addressed.

Considerations for feeding alternative protein-based diets

Healthy dogs and cats

Provided that the diet meets all nutritional aims, there should be no specific considerations for feeding this type of diet to healthy dogs and cats. Confirmation of nutritional adequacy would require good formulation, diet analysis and properly conducted feeding trials (see Chapter 3).

Dogs and cats with various diseases

Soya beans are already commonly used in dietetic food. Other protein sources such as insect-based proteins are likely to follow; however, they have only recently started being used in pet food production.

Provided that they demonstrate clinical efficacy, insect-based proteins could offer a viable choice for dietetic food in the future.

Feeding alternative protein-based diets in a hospital environment

There are no specific considerations for a patient fed an alternative protein-based diet in a hospital environment provided that it does not pose a risk to any other patients or staff.

Conclusion

Alternative protein-based diets might offer a new, potentially more sustainable choice for pet owners concerned about the environmental impact of using animal proteins in food. These diets could become a common choice in the future.

References and further reading

Alexander P, Berri A, Moran D, Reay D and Rounsevell MDA (2020) The global environmental paw print of pet food. *Global and Environmental Change* **65**, 102153

Areerat S, Chundang P, Lekcharoensuk C and Kovitvadhi A (2021) Possibility of using house cricket (*Acheta domesticus*) or mulberry silkworm (*Bombyx mori*) pupae meal to replace poultry meal in canine diets based on health and nutrient digestibility. *Animals* **11**, 2680

Bajuk BP, Zrimšek P, Kotnik T, Leonardi A, Križaj I and Strajn BJ (2021) Insect protein-based diet as potential risk of allergy in dogs. *Animals* **11(7)**, 1942

Case LP, Carey DP, Hirakawa DA and Daristotle L (2000) *Canine and Feline Nutrition: A Resource for Companion Animals Professionals*, 2nd edn. Mosby, St Louis

FEDIAF (2022) *Novel food*. [Available: https://www.efsa.europa.eu/en/topics/topic/novel-food]

Freel TA, McComb A and Koutsos EA (2021) Digestibility and safety of dry black soldier fly larvae meal and black soldier fly larvae oil in dogs. *Journal of Animal Science* **99**

Jeffers JG, Shanley KJ and Meyer EK (1991) Diagnostic testing of dogs for food hypersensitivity. *Journal of the American Veterinary Medical Association* **198**, 245–250

Kasimanickam V, Kasimanickam M and Kasimanickam R (2021) Antibiotics use in food animal production: escalation of antimicrobial resistance – where are we now in combating AMR? *Medical Sciences* **9**, 14

McCusker S, Buff PR, Yu Z and Fascetti AJ (2014) Amino acid content of selected plant, algae and insect species: a search for alternative protein sources for use in pet foods. *Journal of Nutritional Science* **3**, e39

Meneguz M, Shiavone A, Gai F *et al.* (2018) Effect of rearing substrate on growth performance, waste reduction efficiency and chemical composition of black soldier fly (*Hermetia illucens*) larvae. *Journal of the Science of Food Agriculture* **98**, 5776–5784

Norton RD, Lenox CE, Manino P and Vulgamott JC (2016) Nutritional considerations for dogs and cats with liver disease. *Journal of the American Animal Hospital Association* **52**, 1–7

Ramos-Elorduy BJ (1997) The importance of edible insects in the nutrition and economy of people of the rural areas of Mexico. *Ecology of Food Nutrition* **36**, 347–366

Ritchie H and Roser M (2021) Soy. *Our World in Data*. [Available from: https://ourworldindata.org/soy]

Smith CE, Parnell LD, Lai CQ, Rush JE and Freeman LM (2021) Investigation of diets associated with dilated cardiomyopathy in dogs using foodomics analysis. *Scientific Reports* **11**, 1–12

Spranghers T, Ottoboni M, Klootwijk C *et al.* (2017) Nutritional composition of black soldier fly (*Hermetia illucens*) prepupae reared on different organic waste substrates. *Journal of the Science of Food Agriculture* **97**, 2594–2600

Stein HH, Berger LL, Drackley JK, Fahey GC, Hernot DC and Parsons CM (2008) Nutritional properties and feeding values of soybeans and their coproducts. In: *Soybeans, Chemistry, Production, Processing and Utilization*, ed. LA Johnson, PJ White and R Galloway, pp. 613–660. AOCS Press, Illinois

Online extras

This chapter includes:

● **A client information leaflet that is available to download and print from the BSAVA Library**

Access via QR code or: bsavalibrary.com/nutrition_8

Pre-conception, gestation and lactation

9

The creation of new life in all mammals is nutritionally challenging. Therefore, health status of a female before conception should not be overlooked since it can affect fetal development, parturition and also future development of neonates. Once fertilization has occurred, physiological adaptations arise early in cats, meaning there are nutritional pressures throughout gestation; in contrast, with dogs there is little change in nutritional requirements until the third trimester. An optimal nutritional recommendation is central to the health of both the dam and offspring. Following parturition, lactation creates one of the most nutritionally challenging states that most female mammals experience and optimal nutrition is paramount if they are to successfully raise and protect their young. Careful consideration and frequent review of the nutrition provided must be recommended from the time prior to conception through to the end of lactation to ensure the health of all.

Pre-conception

This is a key period before mating and, to ensure optimal development of the fetus, both dam and sire should:
- Have an ideal weight and condition (e.g. body condition score (BCS) 4–5/9 for dogs, 5–6/9 for cats)
  - An underweight BCS may significantly reduce the chances of conception and might even mean that conception is not possible.
- Be in a good state of physical fitness
- Be free from disease, including hereditary diseases
  - Many health screening schemes and deoxyribonucleic acid (DNA) testing schemes are available (e.g. hip scoring) to check for some of the more common problems.
- Have a good temperament with no significant behavioural concerns
- Not be closely related
  - Calculators are available for pedigree dogs to determine the degree of inbreeding.

Gestation

This is the period of fetal development following implantation of a fertilized egg.

Gestation for dogs = 63–65 days
Gestation for cats = approximately 65 days

When the dam is not in ideal bodyweight at the time of conception, there can be detrimental effects during gestation. Underweight dams, or those in poor health, have a reduced fertility capability, litters are typically smaller, and lighter neonate birth weights are then common. Compromised lactation is often observed in these cases, increasing the chances that hand rearing might be required (see Chapter 10), all of which can predispose to poorer neonate survival (Schroeder and Smith, 1994). Conversely, when the dam is in overweight or obese body condition, a smaller litter size of large fetuses can result, increasing the risk of dystocia and with a greater chance that a Caesarean section might be required (Lawler and Monti, 1984).

Lactation

Following parturition, the production of milk by the dam will sustain the life of the neonates by providing all nutrients and fluids until weaning. Weaning commences at 3–4 weeks of age, with full nutritional and behavioural weaning completed by 8–12 weeks of age. Maternal milk is species-specific, containing amounts of fat, protein, calcium and fluid to meet the needs of the growing puppies or kittens (see Chapter 10); milk from other species should not be given other than for short-term use in emergency situations.

Lactation not only provides complete nutrition for neonates but, within the first 48 hours, delivers passive immunity to the neonate in the form of essential immunoglobulins. Unlike humans, where 80% of maternal antibodies are transferred via the placenta, only 10–20% pass via this route in dogs and cats. These species rely on the colostrum (first milk) during the first few hours after birth to deliver immune protection. Protection from maternal antibodies lasts until approximately 16 weeks of age, by which time most vaccination programmes will have commenced, thereby stimulating acquired immunity.

Essential elements

Pre-conception

Before gestation, both dams and sires should ideally have a good bodyweight and be in ideal body condition (Yang-Fei J et al., 2018; Sones and Balogh, 2023). This can be achieved by feeding suitable diets in the correct portions, limited quantities of treats, frequent monitoring and adjustments throughout adulthood. Should either of the potential parents be underweight, overweight or obese before conception, acheiving an ideal weight is recommended (see Chapter 15).

Gestation

In both cats and dogs, food consumption may decrease just before and shortly after parturition but will rapidly increase again as large quantities of additional energy are needed for lactation.

Dogs

During gestation, the pregnant dam (Figure 9.1) should initially be fed either a complete and balanced diet suitable for adults or a diet purpose-formulated to meet the needs of a dam during gestation. Food formulated for growth (i.e. puppy food) can be fed in the last trimester due to its greater energy density. The greatest nutritional consideration during gestation, which lasts for approximately 8 weeks, is energy requirement; in the initial weeks, the energy requirement is similar to standard adult maintenance energy requirement and, therefore, no dietary changes are required. However, in the last third of gestation, the dam will require an additional 15–25% (depending on litter size) of energy above maintenance requirements (Fontaine, 2012). Feeding in multiple meals is usually recommended because feeding volume will increase to facilitate this additional energy intake. More frequent smaller meals will limit stomach and intestinal 'fill', ensuring that there is sufficient abdominal space for the fetuses to grow. This is of particular concern when the litter size is large.

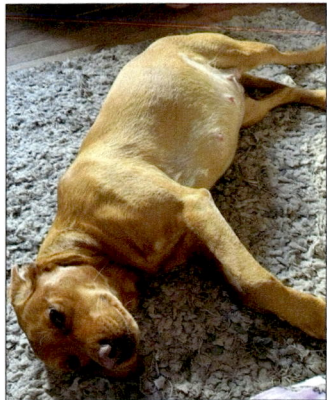

Figure 9.1: Female Labrador Retriever during gestation.
(Courtesy of Louise Dale)

Cats

In contrast, cats tend to lose weight during lactation and, as a result, they must accumulate adipose tissue reserves during gestation (Figure 9.2). Therefore, immediately following conception, it is recommended that pregnant queens be fed 10% additional food, to prepare them for the changes that will occur post-partum (Loveridge and Rivers, 1989). As with bitches, multiple small meals are recommended. Food consumption may decrease just before and shortly after giving birth but will rapidly increase again as large quantities of additional energy is needed for lactation.

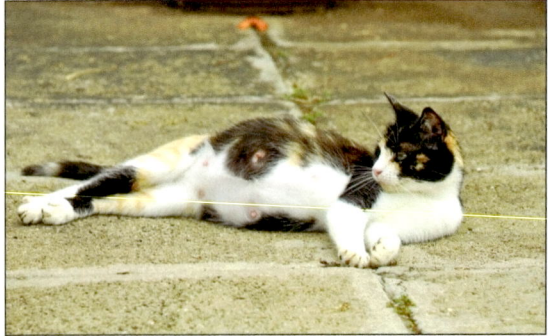

Figure 9.2: Female tortoiseshell cat during gestation.
(Image used under licence from Shutterstock.com ©Paul McKinnon)

Additional nutrients

Folic acid (Domoslawska *et al.*, 2013) and docosahexaenoic acid (DHA) (Dahms *et al.*, 2019) are required during gestation for fetal neural tube development and to reduce the risk of cleft palate, as well as facilitating growth of the fetal brain and retina. Diets formulated for gestation should be fortified with these nutrients. Contrary to the belief of some breeders, supplementation with calcium is not required. Additional calcium may cause skeletal deformities and increase the chances of eclampsia (Forsberg and Eneroth, 2010). Provided that a complete and balanced diet is being fed, no supplementation is required.

Lactation

For reproducing females, lactation overwhelmingly has the greatest energy requirements (Figure 9.3). If the diet does not meet energy needs, there will be rapid mobilization of energy from existing stores (e.g. adipose tissue), leading to weight loss which, if severe, could have a negative effect on health. Precise energy needs are difficult to ascertain as they are affected by the health status of the dam and the litter size (Figure 9.4). To address this, and to maximize the opportunity for sufficient energy intake, *ad libitum* feeding is recommended. Given that milk is comprised of 80% water, an abundant water supply must be offered throughout lactation.

Weeks following parturition	Energy requirements of the lactating bitch or queen
1	1.5–2 x MER
2	2 x MER
3	2.5–3 x MER
4	2.5–3 x MER
4+	As weaning commences energy requirements will reduce back to MER by the time all the young have left to go to their new homes, or when the mother refuses to allow her young to feed

Figure 9.3: Increase in maintenance energy requirement (MER) for lactating females.
(Data from National Research Council, 2006)

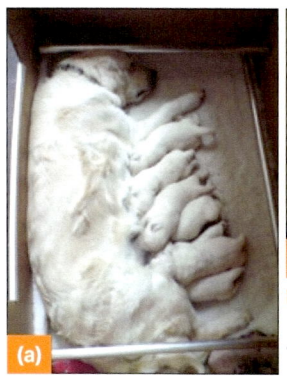

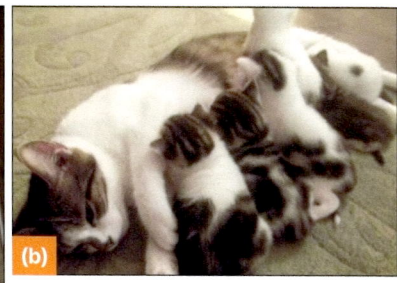

Figure 9.4: Lactation has the greatest energy requirements for reproducing (a) dogs and (b) cats. Energy requirements can be affected by the health status of the dam and the size of the litter.
(© Georgia Woods-Lee)

Suitable diet choices

Given that the nutritional demands of reproduction are so great, particularly during gestation and lactation, diets should be readily digestible and energy dense to ensure that the volume of food per meal is reasonably small. Commercial products formulated to be suitable are labelled 'for use during gestation/lactation' or 'for all life stages'; appropriately formulated diets for growing animals may be suitable choices during lactation. Commercial dry foods typically have approximately 10% moisture content and, therefore, are energy dense. These make a suitable choice, enabling feeding in smaller quantities, although a large feeding amount is still likely required. In contrast, commercial wet foods are less suitable because the greater water content (approximately 80%) and lower energy density make it hard to meet energy requirements with the required food volume, although these do help provide needed moisture. Home-prepared cooked diets (see Chapter 5) can be used provided that they are formulated and overseen by an appropriately qualified person (see Chapter 1). Compared with dry foods, these diets usually have a relatively high moisture content and are less energy dense. Given the risks of pathogenic infection, raw meat-based diets (see Chapter 6) are not recommended at any time during gestation, lactation or growth.

Communication with pet owners

Whether experienced or new to the breeding of cats and dogs, owners will be excited at the prospect of rearing puppies and kittens and therefore be motivated to make appropriate choices about diet. This provides the veterinary professional with an excellent opportunity to advise on suitable diet choices and approaches to feeding, as well as correcting any practices that might be detrimental to the dam and offspring. Further, it is important that pet owners know who to contact if any aspects of pre-conception, gestation and parturition do not go as planned.

Conclusion

Planning for a healthy gestation and lactation are key to producing healthy neonates, with nutrition playing a key role in supporting the dam throughout this time. The pre-conception, gestation and post-parturition periods present different nutritional challenges and, as a result, working closely with pet owners and recommending dynamic nutritional plans will be essential for the health of both the dam and offspring.

References and further reading

Dahms I, Bailey-Hall E, Sylvester E *et al.* (2019) Safety of a novel feed ingredient, Algal Oil containing EPA and DHA, in a gestation-lactation-growth feeding study in Beagle dogs. *PLoS One* **14**, e0217794

Domosławska A, Jurczak A and Janowski T (2013) Oral folic acid supplementation decreases palate and/or lip cleft occurrence in Pug and Chihuahua puppies and elevates folic acid blood levels in pregnant bitches. *Polish Journal of Veterinary Science* **16**, 33–37

Fontaine E (2012) Food intake and nutrition during pregnancy, lactation and weaning in the dam and offspring. *Reproduction in Domestic Animals* **47**, 326–330

Forsberg CL and Eneroth A (2010) Abnormalities in pregnancy, parturition, and the periparturient period. *Textbook of Veterinary Internal Medicine*, 7th edn. Elsevier Saunders, Missouri

Jia YF, Feng Q, Ge ZY *et al.* (2018) Obesity impairs male fertility through long-term effects on spermatogenesis. *BMC Urology* **18**, 42

Kennel Club (2025) *Breeding resources and health schemes*. [Available from: https://www.thekennelclub.org.uk/health-and-dog-care/what-we-do-for-dog-health/breeding-resources-and-health-schemes/]

Kennel Club (2025) *Inbreeding coefficient lookup*. [Available from: https://www.thekennelclub.org.uk/search/inbreeding-co-efficient/]

Lawler DF and Monti KL (1984) Morbidity and mortality in neonatal kittens. *American Journal of Veterinary Research* **45**, 1455–1459

Loveridge GG and Rivers JPW (1989) Body weight changes and energy intakes of cats during pregnancy and lactation. *Nutrition of the Dog and Cat: Waltham Symposium* **7**, 113–132

National Research Council (2006) *Nutrient Requirements of Dogs and Cats*. The National Academies Press, Washington DC

Royal Canin (2024) *Feline and Canine Paediatric Care*. [Available from: https://vetportal.royalcanin.co.uk/news/new-practical-guide-for-veterinarians]

Schroeder GE and Smith GA (1994) Food intake and growth of German Shepherd puppies. *Journal of Small Animal Practice* **35**, 587–591

Sones J and Balogh O (2023) Body condition and fertility in dogs. *Veterinary Clinics of North America: Small Animal Practice* **53(5)** 1031–1045

 Online extras

This chapter includes:

● A client information leaflet that is available to download and print from the BSAVA Library

Access via QR code or: 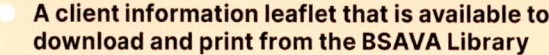 bsavalibrary.com/nutrition_9

Kittens and puppies

10

From the moment kittens and puppies are born, nutrition is vital for their growth and health. Therefore, it is crucial to understand the different elements of feeding kittens and puppies throughout the growth period and into adulthood. The growth period spans from the time of birth to the age at which skeletal maturity is reached (Figure 10.1).

Species	Age at skeletal maturity
Cats	9–12 months
Small dog breeds	8–12 months
Medium dog breeds	12–18 months
Large and giant dog breeds	18–24 months

Figure 10.1: Age at which puppies and kittens reach skeletal maturity.

Nutritional considerations for feeding neonates from birth until weaning

The term 'neonate' describes the first 2 weeks of life, with the first 36 hours being the most critical. Kittens and puppies are born altricial (helpless), relying on their mother for food, water and warmth, as well as to urinate and defecate (triggered by perineal stimulation).

Kittens and puppies reared by the queen or bitch

In most instances, newborn kittens and puppies feed exclusively on maternal milk for the first 3–4 weeks. In the first 48 hours post-partum, lactating queens and bitches produce colostrum. This not only provides neonates with hydration but also passive immunity by transfer of immunoglobulins through the intestinal mucosa, providing protection until the development of acquired immunity following vaccination. Unlike humans, where most passive immunity (80%) is passed via the placenta, in kittens and puppies 80–90% of passive immunity is derived from the colostrum (Delaney and Fascetti, 2023). The nutritional requirements of kittens and puppies change during the first 3–4 weeks of life and this is reflected in the composition of maternal milk, with increased amounts of both protein and lactose being observed during this time (Adkins *et al.*, 2001).

Like all mammalian neonates, kittens and puppies feed on demand. As the stomach is small, they must feed often and in small amounts to satisfy nutritional needs. Typically, kittens and puppies feed hourly during the first week of life, with the intervals between feeding extending gradually as they grow (see Figure 10.3). After feeding, kittens and

---

puppies should sleep. If they are vocal and generally unsettled, this can indicate hunger or discomfort. In these cases, the milk supply may be compromised and assessment of maternal milk will be required. Where milk production is poor or absent, supplementary feeding with a commercial milk replacement will be required (Delaney and Fascetti, 2023). In addition, some breeds of dog can have very large litters (e.g. >12 puppies). In these cases, the mother is unlikely to successfully feed all the puppies sufficiently, so supplementary feeding with a milk replacement product may be required. It is important that all puppies within the litter are provided with maternal milk (particularly the colostrum) alongside the milk replacement product to ensure immunity.

Kittens and puppies reared by hand

In rare situations, maternal milk may not be available. The lack of maternal milk can be due to poor or absent milk production caused by low bodyweight and poor overall condition of the dam, rejection or abandonment of the kittens or puppies, or death of the bitch or queen. If possible, kittens and puppies should be transferred to a foster mother if a suitable one is available; if not, then a milk replacement formula will be required. It is important to note that the nutrient composition of maternal milk differs between species (Figure 10.2) and this should be considered when selecting a replacement formula (Adkins et al., 1997; Zottman et al., 1997).

Nutrient	Milk composition of different species			
	Cat	Dog	Cow	Goat
Metabolizable energy (ME) (kcal/100 g)	121	146	64	69
Crude protein (g/100 g)	7.5	7.5	3.3	3.6
Crude fat (g/100 g)	8.5	9.5	3.6	4.1
Moisture (g/100 g)	79	77.3	87.7	84.2
Lactulose (g/100 g)	4.0	3.3	4.7	4.0
Calcium (g/100 g)	180	240	119	133

Figure 10.2: Comparison of nutrient compositions of milk from different species.
(Debraekeleer et al., 2000)

Hand-rearing kittens and puppies is a challenging task, but can be one of the most rewarding. To successfully hand rear fully orphaned kittens and puppies, the carer must mimic the care normally provided by the bitch or queen, including adopting a suitable feeding regimen (Figure 10.3). An optimal environmental temperature should be provided (18 to 27°C); this can be achieved using a heat source (e.g. a heat pad or lamp; Figure 10.4) placed at one end of the enclosure. There should be a temperature gradient within the closure, thereby allowing kittens and puppies to regulate their own body temperature. Heat pads and lamps should be regularly inspected to ensure that they are not becoming too hot and at risk of burning the kittens or puppies. Kittens and puppies also require a degree of humidity in the environment. Dry environments (often caused by air conditioning) should be avoided, if possible; alternatively, a small room humidifier can be used to humidify the immediate environment. In addition, the carer should stimulate urination and defecation after each meal by gently rubbing the perineal region in a circular motion using damp, warm cotton wool.

Age	Approximate feeding frequency
1–2 weeks old	Every 2 hours
2–3 weeks old	Every 3 hours
3–4 weeks old	Every 4–5 hours
4 weeks old	Start weaning

Figure 10.3: Feeding regime for hand-rearing neonates.

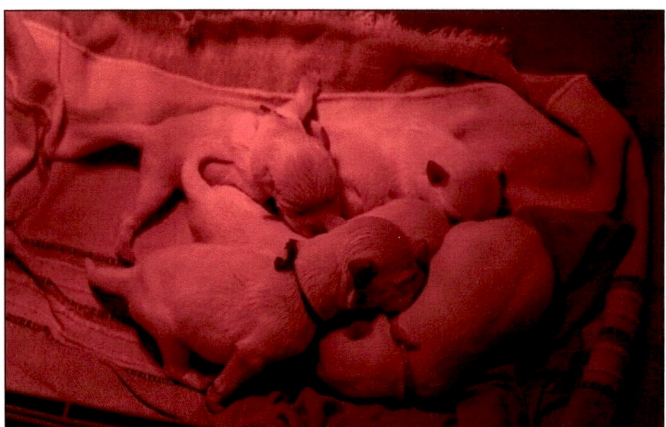

Figure 10.4: Newborn puppies under an infrared heat lamp.
(Image used under the licence from Shutterstock.com © Pawparazzi88)

Excessive bedding should not be provided within the enclosure because kittens and puppies might become trapped and then suffocate. The type of bedding should also be considered. Bedding designed for veterinary patients is ideal as it is soft, retains warmth and can help soak up any bodily fluids or spilt food, thus preventing the kittens and puppies from becoming wet and cold. Blankets that have an open weave or knit should be avoided, as small legs or nails can become stuck and injuries occur. When feeding, care should be taken to avoid inundating the kitten or puppy with milk as this increases the risk of aspiration pneumonia. Specifically designed feeding bottles (Figure 10.5) can help prevent this from occurring, although the flow of milk should be monitored and adjusted accordingly. Overfeeding should be avoided as this may cause diarrhoea. Strict hygiene routines should always be employed with careful washing of all equipment used for feeding in order to reduce the risk of illness.

Expected weight gain

Kittens should gain a minimum of 100 g per week until 6 months of age (Lawler and Bebiak, 1986; Gross *et al.*, 2010). Puppies weight gain should be measured as a percentage increase of their current weight each week (Figure 10.6). Daily weighing of kittens (Figure 10.7) and puppies, particularly those that are being hand reared, is advisable to ensure that they are gaining weight consistently. Failure to gain weight for even 1 day is a cause for concern and further investigations are required to determine the cause.

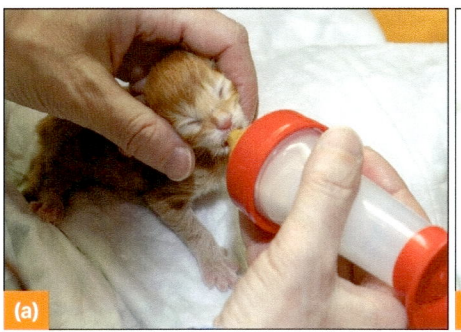
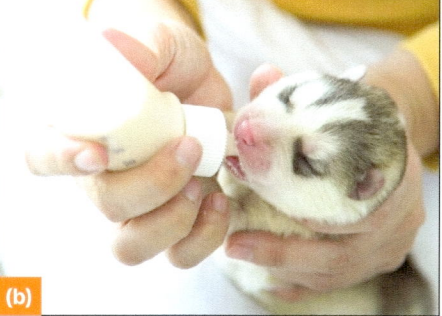

Figure 10.5: Feeding (a) a kitten and (b) a puppy using specifically designed feeding bottles.
(Images used under the licence from Shutterstock.com © (a) Vikentiy Elizarov; (b) Anucha Pongpatimeth)

Age	Percentage gain of current bodyweight
1 week	8
2 weeks	6
3 weeks	4
4 weeks	3.5

Figure 10.6: Percentage weekly weight gain for puppies.
(Debraekeleer *et al.*, 2000)

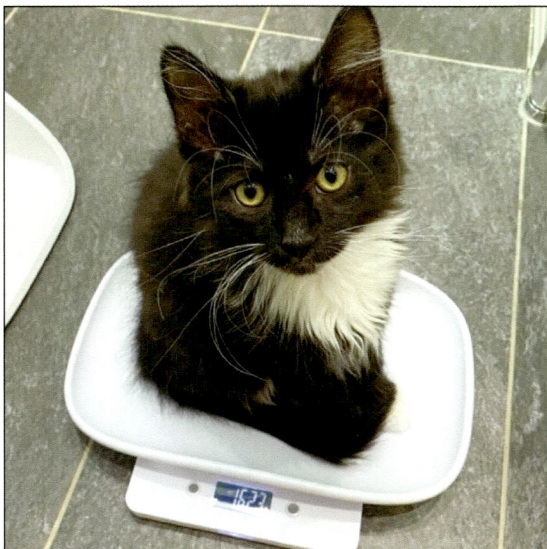

Figure 10.7: Weighing a kitten on digital scales.
(© Georgia Woods-Lee)

Pre-weaning mortality

Pre-weaning mortality rates have been reported as up to 13% in kittens (Dolan *et al.*, 2021) and 15% in puppies (Lawler, 2008); although it should be noted that neonatal mortality can be substantially higher at around 40%. Nutrition plays a key role in preventing these deaths, with the first 36 hours of life being the most critical. If high mortality rates occur, the possible causes including poor nutrition should always be investigated.

Nutritional considerations for feeding kittens and puppies from weaning onwards

Weaning

At 3–4 weeks of age, the digestive system has matured sufficiently to allow kittens and puppies to consume soft, solid foods. During the weaning process, there should be a gradual switch from a liquid to a solid food diet (Figure 10.8). Although this is often a messy process, kittens and puppies typically adapt quickly and the transition to a prepared pet food can be complete by 6 weeks of age. Many of the deciduous teeth will also have erupted by this time. It should be noted that even though nutritional weaning can be complete by 6 weeks of age, if the mother is still spending time with and caring for the young, they will continue to consume maternal milk. Further, since behavioural weaning can take up to 8 weeks, breeders should be encouraged to allow the mother and young to stay together until the kittens or puppies are ready to be rehomed. Kittens that nurse for 7 weeks or longer are less likely to become overweight adult cats (van Lent *et al.*, 2021).

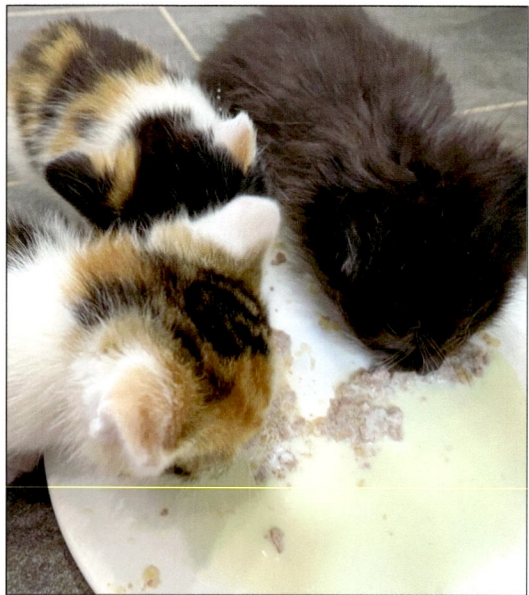

Figure 10.8: Kittens should be gradually introduced to solid food. In the first instance, a mixture of wet food and milk replacement formula should be provided.
(© Georgia Woods-Lee)

Transitioning to a new home

At approximately 8 weeks of age, many kittens and puppies will be rehomed. For some pedigree kittens, rehoming may occur later (e.g. at 16 weeks), with vaccination and neutering often being undertaken before the kittens leave the breeder. Once rehomed, the diet will often be changed to a food type preferred by the new owner; however, since being taken from their stable birth environment can be challenging (both physically and emotionally), breeders should inform the new owners of the specific diet brand and type of food the kitten or puppy is currently consuming or provide the owner with some of this food. This food should be used initially and can also help facilitate a gradual transition to a new diet, if necessary. Such a gradual transition facilitates acceptance by the kitten or puppy, while also minimizing the risk of gastric disturbances developing as a result of the dietary change (see Chapter 18).

Suitable diet choices

The most suitable diet to feed growing kittens and puppies is one that is specifically designed for their life stage. Since nutrient requirements change rapidly throughout the growth phase, the feeding quantity should be regularly checked alongside bodyweight, ideally with reference to a growth chart (this is particularly important for large- and giant-breed puppies; see below). Good quality diets, formulated for growth, will provide guidance on the packaging to ensure good feeding practices are followed.

Meal frequency

At the time of weaning, the queen or bitch is likely to still allow her young to feed, although this will become less frequent as they start to spend more time away from their offspring. Therefore, solid food can be offered at a frequency of 4–6 meals per day, with the number of meals gradually reducing and the intervals between meals increasing as the kittens and puppies grow. Multiple meals are preferred because of the smaller stomach capacity of kittens and puppies (compared with adult cats and dogs), to ensure that sufficient food is consumed to meet energy and other nutritional requirements. Depending on the food type provided (e.g. wet or dry), the feeding volume will differ, and this may inform how many meals are needed for sufficient food to be consumed each day.

Feeding quantity

Although many calculations exist for estimating a feeding quantity for kittens and puppies throughout the growth period, pragmatically, owners should be advised to use the feeding guide on the food packaging as a starting point. If dry food is used, portions should be weighed out on digital scales to ensure accuracy. The amount fed can be adjusted according to response, preferably by regularly weighing and monitoring the growth pattern using a growth chart. Bodyweight should be measured at least every month until 6 months of age, then at least every 2–3 months (but more often if possible), and the feeding quantity adjusted as required. In addition to monitoring bodyweight, body condition score (BCS) can also be assessed (see Chapter 15), although caution should be exercised because methods have not been fully validated in growing kittens and puppies. Nonetheless, this technique can help to confirm decisions based on weight change.

Misconceptions about feeding kittens and puppies

Any diet can be fed to a kitten or puppy

Only diets that have been specifically formulated to be suitable for the growth phase should be fed. Attempting to use alternative diet types can be challenging, especially because nutrient and energy demands are greatest during growth. Home-prepared cooked diets could be considered (see Chapter 5), but only if the recipe is developed by someone with a suitable qualification who will ensure nutritional adequacy and safety (see Chapter 3). Kittens, as obligate carnivores, require diets containing ingredients from animal sources to provide complete nutrition. Recently, trends of feeding vegetarian or vegan diets to cats have increased in popularity; however, it is unclear whether such diets are suitable for kittens and their use is not currently advised (see Chapter 7).

Kittens and puppies should be allowed to eat as much as they want

As neonates, kittens and puppies can, and should, be fed on demand and this pattern should be mimicked as closely as possible if hand-rearing. From weaning onwards, the feeding quantity should usually be limited and it is not advisable to allow most kittens and puppies to feed *ad libitum* as over consumption can occur. Given that obesity is prevalent in adult cats and dogs, pet owners need to regulate food intake throughout life (German *et al.*, 2018; Association for Pet Obesity Prevention, 2022).

Large- and giant-breed puppies

Dogs as a species are unique within the animal kingdom due to the huge variety in their size. For large- and giant-breed puppies, their size is associated with particular nutritional considerations. These breeds have an extended growth phase (Figure 10.9) and must be fed a complete and balanced diet throughout this period to promote optimal growth. A suitable diet provides:

- Careful energy intake (due to being lower in fats)
- Sufficient protein
- Sufficient calcium – supplementation is not required at any stage. Calcium supplements can increase the risk of developing orthopaedic diseases (Dämmrich, 1991).

Size of breed	Adult weight	Age at end of extended growth phase
Large	>25 kg	18 months
Giant	>40 kg	18–24 months

Figure 10.9: Age of large- and giant-breed dogs at the end of the extended growth phase.

A switch to a suitable adult diet should not be made before skeletal maturity is reached at the end of the extended growth period. Should a puppy be switched to an adult diet before the end of the growth phase, they will have to consume a larger volume of food to meet their energy and other nutritional needs. In addition, since adult diets are not suitably balanced for puppies, the amount of calcium consumed may also be more than is required. Excessive food intake artificially accelerates growth, increasing the risk of developmental orthopaedic disorders (Lauten, 2006). In fact, approximately 20% of orthopaedic conditions are related to diet (Hazewinkel *et al.*, 2006). These may include:

- Osteochondritis dissecans (OCD)
- Hip dysplasia
- Hypertrophic osteodystrophy.

Communication with pet owners

When a pet owner first brings home a kitten or puppy, they will very quickly form a close bond, and the health of that individual will be paramount. At this time, there will be many factors that owners need to consider and for veterinary professionals to discuss, including:

- Vaccinations
- Endoparasite and ectoparasite control
- Litter tray/toilet training
- Play activity and the use of suitable toys
- Behaviour and training (including socialization and habituation)
- Monitoring growth
- Dental care
- Diet
- Neutering
- Microchipping
- Insurance.

It is vital that nutrition is not forgotten amongst all other considerations as this directly impacts growth and health. Sufficient time should be devoted to enable discussions to be held about correct nutrition and monitoring; utilization of the whole team is recommended. Veterinary nurses are often ideally placed to provide this information to owners. Pet owners will often be highly motivated at this time to seek information and act on advice; therefore, discussions about nutrition should not be delayed.

It is important to stress that there should be no changes to the diet for the first 1–3 days. The owner should obtain information from the breeder about the diet that has been fed and continue this while the kitten or puppy settles into their new home. Any food changes after this point should be made gradually to avoid gastrointestinal disturbances (see above). The new diet should be appropriate for the species, breed and growth phase.

Discussions with the owner about the quantity to feed are also important. Most pet foods have guidance on the packaging that details how much should be fed; however, it is paramount that the owner is aware that the amount of food will need to be adjusted as the kitten or puppy grows. Owners should be counselled about the importance of regular weight and growth checks. The frequency of feeding should also be discussed. The owner should be advised to feed meals within a dedicated time, rather than feeding *ad libitum* as this can lead to over consumption and obesity (see Chapter 15). It is common for pet owners to want to feed their kitten or puppy 'up' to give them the best start, but the risks of overfeeding should be addressed. If a pet is overweight by 1 year of age, it will affect their skeletal maturity and they will have an increased risk of being overweight for life. Owners should be given the following advice to help prevent overfeeding:

- Control portions
  - Weigh out every meal or daily allocation
  - Adjust the portion size as the kitten or puppy grows
- Be careful with any treats
  - Use as part of daily allocation (rather than as additional food)

- Meal frequency
  - Usually 3–4 meals should be provided daily
  - Frequency may be reduced as the kitten or puppy grows.

Preventing obesity during the growth phase

Preventing obesity relies upon two main approaches: limiting calorie intake and monitoring.

Limiting calorie intake

For kitten and puppy owners, one of the best ways of limiting calorie intake is to develop good habits from the start (Figure 10.10).

Habit	Rationale
Feeding only from a bowl or puzzle feeder	By only providing food via a bowl or puzzle feeder (or pocket during training) it limits the locations kittens and puppies will expect food to come from. Should the owner feed from their own plate or table, the expectation of receiving highly rewarding foods will be created. Food-seeking behaviours will become intensified when the owner is eating. In the author's experience, this pressure often leads to the owner being more likely to provide additional food, increasing overall food consumption
Limiting treats	Treats usually have a high fat content and are used as positive rewards as well as to show love and affection. It can be challenging for owners to provide foods that their kitten or puppy considers to be highly rewarding without adding large quantities of extra calories each day. A good habit would be to limit the number of commercial treats provided and instead use part of the daily allocation of food or low-calorie alternatives such as vegetables (courgette is often well accepted in cats) and fruits
Portioning and accuracy	Using digital scales and weighing out the food allocation into portions each day helps prevent over consumption, which can lead to obesity. As growth requirements change over time, frequent evaluation and accurate adjustments of the feeding portion are needed

Figure 10.10: Good habits to develop to prevent the over consumption of food.

Monitoring using growth charts

Traditionally, bodyweight was used as a means of monitoring growth, although it was difficult to confirm whether the growth pattern was normal. Recently, evidence-based growth standards have been developed, enabling regular weight measurements to be used to determine whether the pattern of growth is as expected (see Figure 10.11) (Salt *et al.*, 2017, 2022). The change in bodyweight of kittens and puppies growing optimally will typically track the centile lines on the growth chart. A growth pattern that deviates either upwards or downwards might indicate a problem and veterinary attention is recommended.

Neutering

Kittens are commonly neutered in the United Kingdom (UK) from as early as 8 weeks old (i.e. during the growth phase). Given the well documented association between neutering and weight gain, bodyweight needs to be monitored regularly (ideally every week) for the first few weeks following the surgical procedure (Salt *et al.*, 2023). It should be noted that the risk of weight gain is less pronounced in male kittens and kittens neutered later during the growth phase (>28 weeks of age).

Should excessive weight gain be observed, the diet should be altered to restore an optimal growth pattern. This might involve reducing the amount of food being fed or switching to a lower energy diet that is still appropriate for the life stage of the animal. Many diets designed for neutered animals that are still in the growth phase are now available; these typically have a reduced energy content compared with a standard growth diet. The use of dietetic weight reduction food is not recommended during the growth phase, since these diets are designed for adult cats and dogs. Instead, the rate of weight gain in kittens and puppies identified as in an overweight condition (BCS >6/9) or those having crossed two or more centile lines on the chart can be slowed, with the aim of ensuring that the growth trajectory decreases by a maximum of one centile unit. Should the kitten or puppy still be overweight by the time they reach adulthood, a formal weight management plan can then be instigated and a dietetic weight loss food would be appropriate (see Chapter 15).

Selecting the correct growth chart: Downloadable kitten and puppy growth charts are available (Figure 10.11). There are separate male and female charts, as well as a range of charts for puppies based on predicted adult bodyweight of the breed (Figure 10.12). Occasionally, the puppy may be in between size categories; in such cases, a chart should be selected where the initial weight is closest to the 50th centile. If the growth pattern is not as expected (i.e. the puppy is healthy and in ideal condition but the chart shows a deviation from the typical growth pattern), then an alternative chart should be selected and the weight measurements replotted.

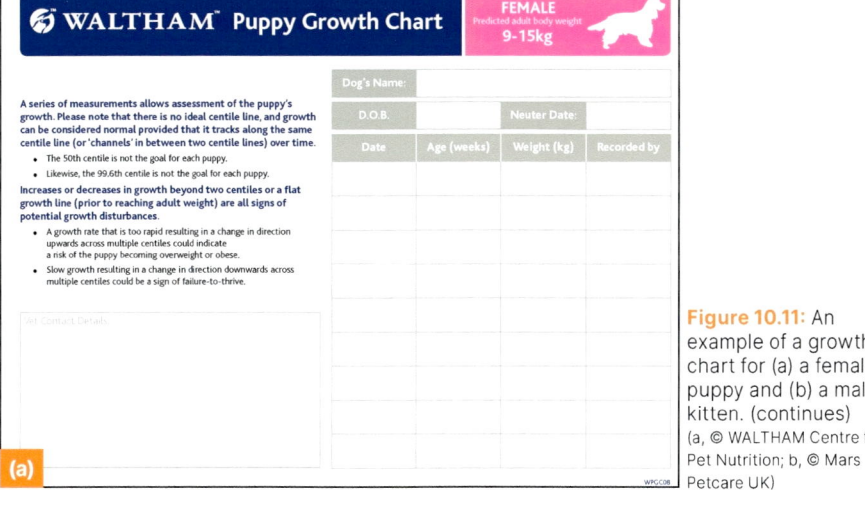

Figure 10.11: An example of a growth chart for (a) a female puppy and (b) a male kitten. (continues) (a, © WALTHAM Centre for Pet Nutrition; b, © Mars Petcare UK)

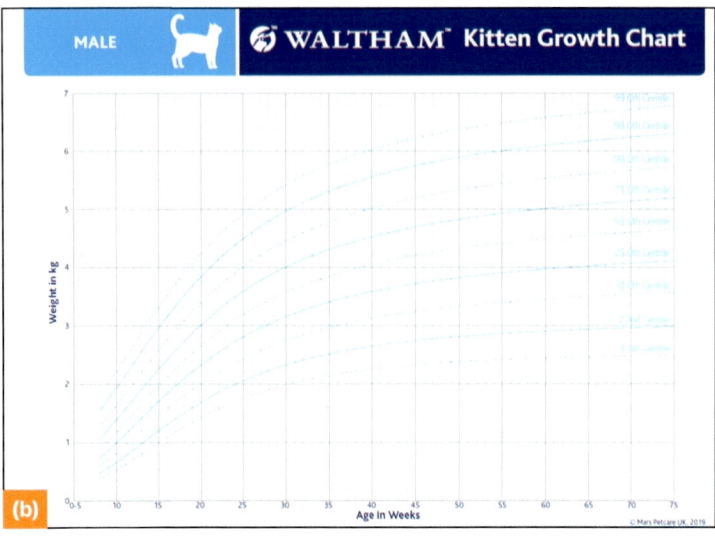

Figure 10.11: continued) An example of a growth chart for (a) a female puppy and (b) a male kitten.

(a, © WALTHAM Centre for Pet Nutrition; b, © Mars Petcare UK)

Plotting measurements on the growth chart: To gather meaningful data on growth, the kitten or puppy should be weighed at least once a month until 6 months of age and then every 2–3 months until skeletal maturity is reached (see above). However, it should be noted that more regular measurements can provide a clearer indication of growth pattern.

1. Weigh the kitten or puppy on suitably sized digital scales after removing any collars or harnesses (see Figure 10.7). Based on date of birth, calculate the age of the animal in weeks.
2. Trace along the X axis (age in weeks) and Y axis (weight in kilograms) of the chart and plot (with a dot or cross) the point where the two intersect.
3. Continue to take weight measurements over time and plot each on the chart. With sufficient measurements, the pattern of growth can be assessed to determine whether it is as expected or is deviating from normal. Growth patterns that require further assessment include:
   a. Crossing centile lines in an upwards direction (especially if two or more lines are crossed)
   b. Crossing centile lines in a downwards direction (especially if two or more lines are crossed)
   c. Recording one or more bodyweight measurement either above or below the most extreme centile lines (i.e. 0.4th centile and 99.6th centile)
   d. Rapid 'catch-up' growth – this is indicated in a kitten or puppy with a weight measurement early in life that is at or below the 0.4th centile that subsequently catches up to a more normal centile.
4. As long as bodyweight measurements are within the area covered by the 0.4th to 99.6th centiles, there is no best or worst centile line to follow; the kitten or puppy should track most closely to the centile that is appropriate for their breed and stature. Once the closest centile line has been determined, trace this line forward to the point of skeletal maturity (approximately 10–12 months of age; see Figure 10.1) to estimate adult bodyweight.

5. Once the kitten or puppy reaches skeletal maturity and body condition has been confirmed to be optimal (based on BCS), record the weight of the animal in the clinical notes as the 'healthy adult weight'.

Predicted adult bodyweight (kg)	Breeds
Less than 6.5	Chihuahua, Maltese, Miniature Pinscher, Pomeranian, Toy Poodle, Yorkshire Terrier
6.5–9	Bichon Frise, Dachshund, Jack Russel Terrier, Lhasa Apso, Miniature Schnauzer, Pekingese, Rat Terrier, Shih Tzu
9–15	American Cocker Spaniel, Beagle, Boston Terrier, Fox Terrier, Pug
15–30	American Shepherd Dog, Basset Hound, Boxer, Chow Chow, English Bulldog, Siberian Husky
30–40	American Bulldog, German Shepherd Dog, Golden Retriever, Labrador Retriever

Figure 10.12: The growth chart selected for monitoring the growth of puppies should be based on the predicted adult bodyweight of the breed.

Conclusion

Feeding an appropriate diet throughout the entire growth phase and dynamically changing the quantities of food based on growth pattern will give kittens and puppies the best start in life. By monitoring bodyweight and tracking growth, optimal growth can be achieved and obesity prevented. Teaching both the pet and owner good feeding habits can help ensure optimal health during the growth phase and throughout adult life.

References and further reading

Adkins Y, Lepine AJ and Lönnerdal B (2001) Changes in protein and nutrient composition of milk throughout lactation in dogs. *American Journal of Veterinary Research* **62(8)**, 1266–1272

Adkins Y, Zicker SC, Lepine A and Lönnerdal B (1997) Changes in nutrient and protein composition of cat milk during lactation. American *Journal of Veterinary Research* **58**, 370–375

Anton C and Beynen (2015) Dry food for cats. Creature Companion **July**, 54–55

Association for Pet Obesity Prevention (2022) *State of U.S. Pet Obesity Report.* [Available from: petobesityprevention.org/]

Case LP, Carey DP, Hirakawa DA and Daristotle L (2000) Energy. In: Canine and Feline Nutrition: *A Resource for Companion Animals Professionals, 2nd edition,* ed. LP Case *et al.,* pp. 5–15. Mosby, USA

Cave N, Delaney SJ and Larsen JA (2023) Nutritional management of gastrointestinal diseases. In: *Applied Veterinary Clinical Nutrition, 2nd edition*, ed. AJ Fascetti *et al.*, pp. 235–298. John Wiley & Sons, Inc., USA

Dämmrich K (1991) Relationship between nutrition and bone growth in large and giant dogs. *Journal of Nutrition* **121**, 114–121

Debraekeleer J, Gross KL and Zicker SC (2000) Feeding nursing and orphaned puppies from birth to weaning. In: *Small Animal Clinical Nutrition*, ed. MS Hand *et al.*, pp. 295–309. Mark Morris Institute, USA

Delaney SJ and Fascetti AJ (2023) Basic nutrition overview. In: *Applied Veterinary Clinical Nutrition*, 2nd edition, ed. AJ Fascetti *et al.*, pp. 8–28. John Wiley & Sons, Inc., USA

Dolan ED, Doyle E, Tran HR and Slater MR (2021) Pre-mortem risk factors for mortality in kittens less than 8 weeks old at a dedicated kitten nursery. *Journal of Feline Medicine and Surgery* **23**, 730–737

German AJ, Woods GRT, Holden SL, Brennan L and Burke C (2018) Dangerous trends in pet obesity. *Veterinary Record* **182**, 25–25

Gross KL, Becvarova I and Debraekeleer J (2010) Feeding nursing and orphaned kittens from birth to weaning. In: *Small Animal Clinical Nutrition*, ed. MS Hand *et al.*, pp. 415–427. Mark Morris Institute, USA

Hazewinkel H (2023) Nutritional management of orthopedic diseases. In: *Applied Veterinary Clinical Nutrition, 2nd edition*, ed. AJ Fascetti *et al.*, pp. 186–234. John Wiley & Sons, Inc., USA

Lauten S D (2006) Nutritional risks to large-breed dogs: from weaning to the geriatric years. *Veterinary Clinics of North America: Small Animal Practice* **36**, 1345–1359

Lawler DF (2008) Neonatal and pediatric care of the puppy and kitten. *Theriogenology* **70**, 384–392

Lawler DF and Bebiak DM (1986) Nutrition and management of reproduction in the cat. *Veterinary Clinics of North America: Small Animal Practice* **16(3)**, 495–519

Salt C, Butterwick RF, Henzel KS and German AJ (2023) Comparison of growth in neutered Domestic Shorthair kittens with growth in sexually-intact cats. *PLoS One* **18(3)**, DOI: 10.1371/journal.pone.0283016

Salt C, German AJ, Henzel KS and Butterwick RF (2022) Growth standard charts for monitoring bodyweight in Domestic Shorthair kittens from the USA. *PLoS One* **17(11)**, DOI: 10.1371/journal.pone.0277531

Salt C, Morris PJ, German AJ *et al.* (2017) Growth standard charts for monitoring bodyweight in dogs of different sizes. *PLoS One* **12(9)**, DOI: 10.1371/journal.pone.0182064

van Lent D, Vernooij JCM, Stolting MM and Corbee RJ (2021) Kittens that nurse 7 weeks or longer are less likely to become overweight adult cats. *Animals (Basel)* **11(12)**, DOI: 10.3390/ani11123434

Waltham (2022) *Waltham downloadable growth charts.* [Available from: waltham.com/resources]

Zottman B, Dobenecker B, Kienzle E, *et al.* (1997) Investigations on milk composition and milk yield in queens [abstract]. In: *Proceedings: The Waltham International Symposium*, Orlando, FL

Online extras

This chapter includes:

- **A client information leaflet that is available to download and print from the BSAVA Library**

Access via QR code or: bsavalibrary.com/nutrition_10

Senior pets

11

Ageing is a time-dependent, biological process that commences shortly after maturity has been reached. Ageing is not a disease, although predictable signs associated with the ageing process are commonly observed. The greater the lifespan, the more influence physiological and environmental stressors have on homeostasis, resulting in the individual being prone to disease and ultimately death (Fascetti and Delaney, 2012). It is assumed that pets reach their senior years during the last third of life (Salt *et al.*, 2022); the age at which this occurs depends on the species and breed, albeit with considerable individual variation (Figures 11.1 and 11.2). As a result, the effects of ageing will differ amongst pets and management should focus on the clinical manifestations of ageing, rather than simply on chronological age. The speed with which the physiological changes of ageing develop depends on the genetics of the pet, veterinary healthcare and the care provided by the owner, and nutrition (Laflamme, 2005). For this reason, all senior pets should be individually assessed and tailored nutrition plans created.

Breed	Median lifespan (years)	Range (years)
Birman	16.1	1–20.7
Siamese	14.2	0.9–21.1
Crossbred	14.0	0–26.7
Maine Coon	11	0.2–19
Ragdoll	10.1	0.9–14.8
Bengal	7.3	0.6–13.7

Figure 11.1: Age at which various cat breeds reach their senior years.

Breed	Median lifespan (years)	Range (years)
Miniature Poodle	14.2	2–19.4
Border Collie	13.7	0.1–19.1
Miniature Dachshund	13.5	2–19.5
Jack Russell Terrier	13.4	0–24
Dalmatian	13.3	0.9–17.2

Figure 11.2: Age at which various dog breeds reach their senior years. (continues) ▶

Breed	Median lifespan (years)	Range (years)
Golden Retriever	12.5	0.1–17.6
Greyhound	10.7	2.5–16.3
Dobermann	9.2	2.1–13
Bulldog	8.4	0.4–15.2
Mastiff	7.1	0–13.8
Great Dane	6.0	0–11
Dogue de Bordeaux	5.5	0–8.8

Figure 11.2: (continued) Age at which various dog breeds reach their senior years.

Monitoring a senior patient

Given that many of the signs of ageing are not overt or obvious to all owners, a monitoring protocol is recommended to ensure the long-term health of senior pets and to allow for early detection of disease. Figure 11.3 details some of the key parameters that can be monitored and recommendations about the minimum frequency that they should be checked. The protocol should take into consideration the presence of existing diseases and the frequency of monitoring adjusted as necessary.

Parameter	Minimum frequency
Bodyweight (on calibrated scales; see textbox)	Every 3 months
Body condition score[a]	Every 6 months or alongside each bodyweight check
Muscle condition score	Every 6 months
Blood pressure	Every 6 months
Biochemistry and haematology (blood test)	Every 6 months
Urine testing	Every 6 months

Figure 11.3: Potential parameters that can be used for monitoring during ageing along with the suggested frequency. [a]For further information, see Chapter 15.

How to calibrate weighing scales

Weighing scales both for dogs and cats are sensitive pieces of equipment. Every time scales are moved (e.g. for cleaning), it causes inaccuracies. Scales should be calibrated regularly (i.e. at least once a week or after each move) to ensure they always measure weight accurately.

Use a test weight

Test weights can be purchased online; however, a brand new bag of pet food can also be used as pet food is weighed very carefully during manufacture. Allowing 0.1–0.2 kg for packaging weight, when placed on the scales the weight on the display should match the weight stated on the bag.

Check the feet of the scales are level and placed on a solid surface

Scales placed on an uneven surface can cause inaccuracies; the scales should not rock when a pet steps on. Thick rubber matting, wooden or carpeted flooring are not suitable surfaces for weighing scales. If the weight on the display does not match the test weight, the scales might be on an unsuitable surface or the feet may no longer be level. These errors should be amended and the 'zero' or 'Tare' button pressed before placing the test weight on them again. If the inaccuracy persists the scales should be sent for repair.

Age-related changes

Commonly observed age-related changes include:

- Changes to body composition resulting from sarcopenia (muscle mass loss) together with potentially increased adipose tissue mass; the bodyweight may remain stable (Freeman, 2018)
- Alterations in energy requirements (Churchill and Eirmann, 2021)
- Reduced kidney function (Bartges, 2012)
- Hair pigment loss due to reduced tyrosinase activity and decreasing melanocyte numbers, resulting in greying fur particularly around the face (Bellows *et al.*, 2015) (Figure 11.4a)

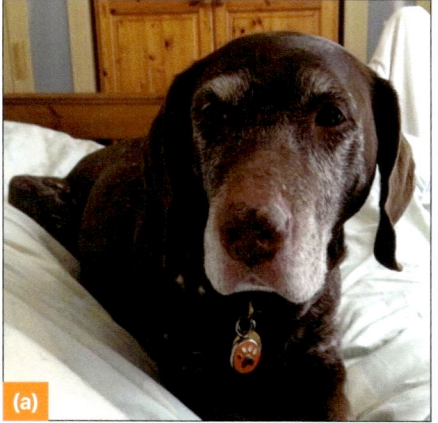 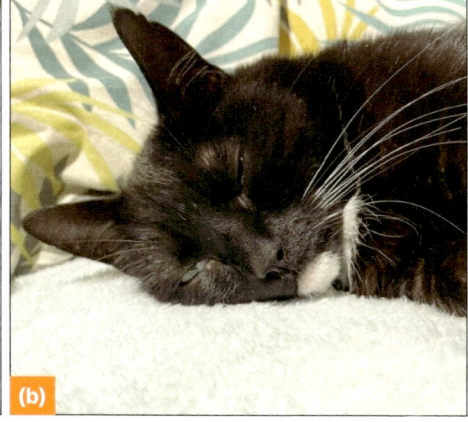

Figure 11.4: Age-related changes seen in dogs and cats include (a) greying of the fur around the head and muzzle and (b) sleeping for an increased amount of time.
(a, Courtesy of Kate Dutton; b, Courtesy of Sam Britton)

- Hair loss due to follicle atrophy (Bellows *et al.*, 2015)
- Reduced ability to groom (Sordo *et al.*, 2020)
- Reduced ability to digest protein and fat (observed in some cats) (Harper, 1998; Stockman, 2024)
- Reduced bone density (McKenzie, 2022)
- Osteoarthritis and associated pain, resulting in decreased appetite and movement (Beale, 2005)
- Reduced cardiovascular function
- Loss of skin elasticity (Bellows *et al.*, 2015; Dhaliwal *et al.*, 2023)
- Reduction in sense perception (e.g. smell, sight, taste – which may affect food intake) (Bellows *et al.*, 2015)
- Reduced cognition (Landsberg and Araujo, 2005)
- Behaviour changes (Landsberg and Araujo, 2005)
- Resisting new routines and environmental changes (Landsberg and Araujo, 2005)
- Increased amounts of sleep (Landsberg *et al.*, 2011) (Figure 11.4b)
- Deteriorating dentition (Lobprise, 2017)
- Decreased sense of thirst (Churchill and Eirmann, 2021).

The effect of nutrition

Optimal nutrition is important to support the needs of dogs and cats as they age. Key nutritional aims include:

- Maintain optimal health
- Delay the effects of ageing (e.g. loss of muscle mass)
- Slow the impact and progression of existing diseases, as well as reduce the risk of new diseases developing
- Extend life expectancy (e.g. in cases of chronic kidney disease (CKD); see Chapter 19)
- Maintain an optimal ('healthy') bodyweight, body condition score (BCS) (see Chapter 15) and muscle condition score (MCS) (Figure 11.5). Although sarcopenia is inevitable, with a suitable diet choice, the effects can be kept to a minimum.

To determine the specific nutritional needs for each pet during the senior life stage, a nutritional assessment is recommended (see Chapter 2) This should be reviewed frequently (e.g. every 4–6 months). Given that ageing is a progressive process, nutritional requirements will change over time, meaning that any plan needs to be dynamic and adaptive. An appropriate nutritional recommendation for senior pets should focus on supporting all metabolic needs, as well as attempting to delay both the onset and progression of chronic diseases prevalent in old age. As with any life stage, nutrition should be complete and balanced with optimal nutrition for senior pets differing from younger adult dogs in several ways.

Essential elements

Energy

The energy requirements of senior pets can be variable. Some pets will remain as active as they were during their adult years well into their senior years; whereas, others will have decreased activity levels, especially if diseases are present that affect mobility (e.g. osteoarthritis, cardiorespiratory disease, obesity), impacting their energy requirements. In general, the energy requirements of cats remain similar throughout adulthood whereas, in dogs, they typically decrease by 18–24% (Harper, 1998). Nonetheless, the specific energy requirement of each pet can only be determined by regularly monitoring bodyweight, BCS and MCS, and tracking changes over time (e.g. 3–4 times per year, or more frequently if another factor or disease is likely to affect the bodyweight). Should the bodyweight alter by more than 5%, action should be taken to either reduce or increase the energy intake, followed by further investigations in the case of unexpected weight loss or monitoring in cases of weight gain.

Obesity in senior pets
One factor that has a significant effect on longevity is an overweight body condition (Salt *et al.*, 2018). Dogs in an overweight condition have a reduced lifespan of between 6 months and 2 years. However, for senior pets in an obese body condition, only modest amounts of weight loss are recommended (e.g. a 15–20% reduction in current bodyweight). This is because significant lean tissue loss usually occurs when >20% of bodyweight is lost and, given that a key nutritional aim is to maintain lean mass, weight loss beyond 20% may be detrimental to the pet. Further, studies in both pets and humans have indicated improved survival rates with a 10–15% increased bodyweight (Lee *et al.*, 2018) when chronic disease is present (e.g. neoplasia, diabetes, heart disease, renal disease; Slupe *et al.*, 2008). This theory is known as the obesity paradox (Armstrong, 2015). Given that controlled weight reduction has many benefits, including improved mobility (Marshall *et al.*, 2010), a modest amount of weight loss can often still be recommended for senior pets with obesity.

Water

Clean, fresh water should always be available to senior pets. Water intake should be monitored periodically (e.g. every 3–4 months). Any unexplained increase in water intake should prompt investigations because it could indicate an underlying disease. In animals with pre-existing conditions causing polydipsia (e.g. CKD, diabetes mellitus, hyperthyroidism), more regular monitoring of water intake might be necessary as adjustments to treatment may be required. As part of the ageing process in cats, the thirst response decreases (Churchill and Eirmann, 2021); therefore, strategies to promote additional fluid intake are recommended to prevent dehydration. Examples of such strategies include the use of water fountains, water sources on all floors of the house for easy access, and the feeding of wet food (which typically contains approximately 80% water).

Protein

Proteins are required throughout the senior life stage for tissue synthesis, immune function and maintenance of lean body mass. There has been much debate about protein restriction for senior cats and dogs to prevent CKD. However, to date, there is no evidence to suggest that this is an effective method for preventing CKD (Ephraim *et al.*, 2020). Avoiding excess phosphorus intake, especially the more soluble forms of phosphorus, is more important for renal health (see below). The sources of protein and phosphorus are often the same, meaning they are very difficult to separate; thus, to reduce phosphorus intake, protein intake must also usually be reduced. In fact, protein requirements increase with age (Cave *et al.*, 2023); lean mass is lost and due to the reduced capacity for protein digestion in many senior cats, protein restriction is not recommended. However, in any senior pet with concurrent CKD, protein intake should be moderated (Elliott *et al.*, 2000) (see Chapter 19).

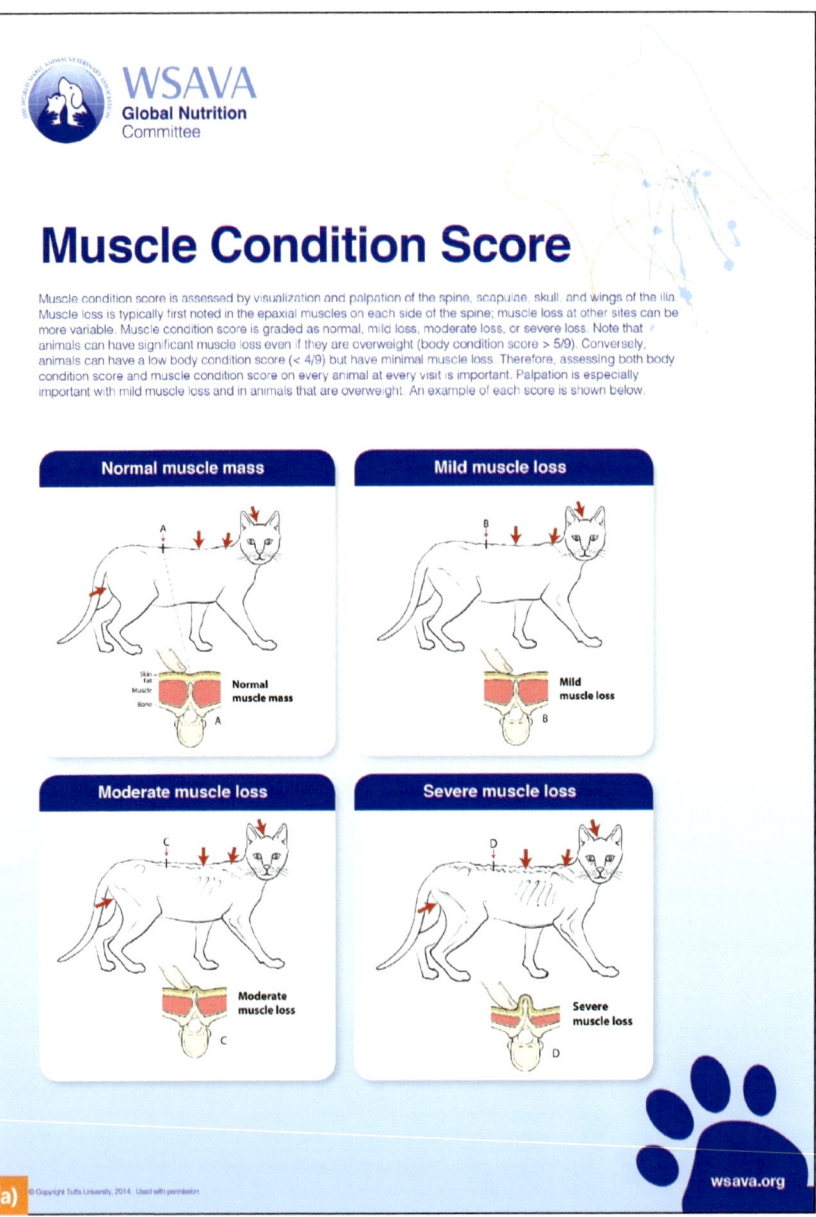

Figure 11.5: Muscle condition scoring systems for (a) cats and (b) dogs. (continues)
(Provided courtesy of the World Small Animal Veterinary Association (WSAVA). Available at the WSAVA Global Nutrition Committee Nutritional Toolkit website: https://wsava.org/global-guidelines/global-nutrition-guidelines/. © Tufts University, 2013; permission requested)

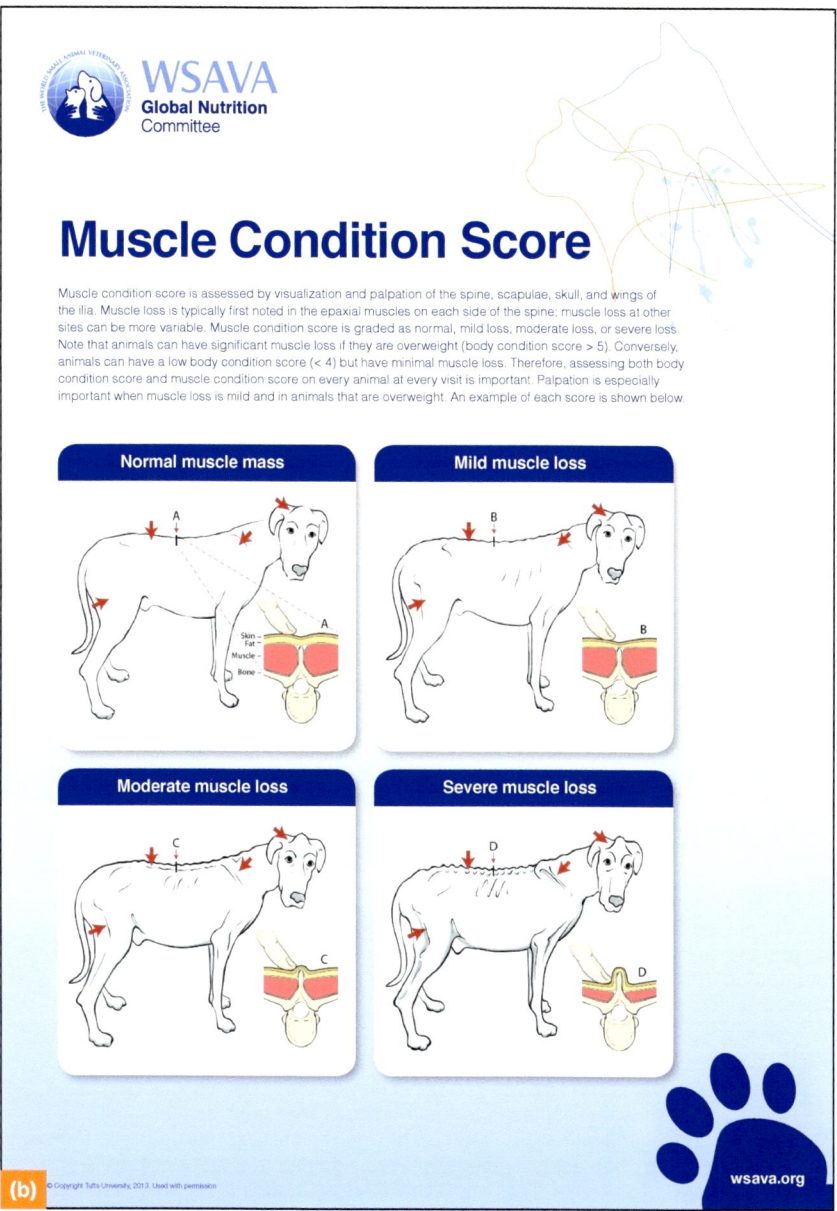

Figure 11.5: (continued) Muscle condition scoring systems for (a) cats and (b) dogs.
(Provided courtesy of the World Small Animal Veterinary Association (WSAVA). Available at the WSAVA Global Nutrition Committee Nutritional Toolkit website: https://wsava.org/global-guidelines/global-nutrition-guidelines/. © Tufts University, 2013; permission requested)

Fat

Fats are an essential part of the diet for ageing pets as they provide energy and essential fatty acids, as well as enhance absorption of fat-soluble vitamins. Fats also increase the palatability of foods, which may be needed to encourage voluntary consumption in senior pets. There is no need to restrict fats in the diet for healthy senior cats and dogs, but care should be taken as large amounts of dietary fat increase energy content and may predispose to obesity.

Carbohydrate

Although not considered to be an essential nutrient for dogs and cats, both can readily utilize dietary carbohydrates, which provide a source of both energy and fibre. By utilizing carbohydrates as an energy source, other nutrients (e.g. proteins) can be spared and used for other vital processes (see above). Adding fibre to the diet of senior pets can also help to maintain gastrointestinal health. Constipation is a common clinical sign in senior pets, especially cats, and they may benefit from dietary fibre supplementation. A balance of fibre types is usually recommended because they have different properties (Figure 11.6). Fermentable fibres (e.g. beet pulp) help nourish the colonocytes by producing short chain fatty acids (e.g. butyrate), whilst non-fermentable fibres (e.g. cellulose) create faecal bulk, promoting good colonic motility. In addition, the gelling effects of fibres such as psyllium are beneficial for cases of constipation. It should be noted that with increased fibre content, the energy density is decreased.

Fibre type and diet composition	Role in the management of constipation
Non-fermentable fibres – increased content in diet	Increases stool bulk and frequency of elimination (Fekete *et al.*, 2004)
Non-fermentable fibres – low content in diet	Increases digestibility of the diet fed. Reduces faecal volume and colonic distension (Fekete *et al.*, 2004)
Digestible fibres (e.g. lactulose) – increased content in diet (Moreno *et al.*, 2022)	Pulls water into the colon to increase the water content of the faeces, which can ease defecation

Figure 11.6: Types of fibre and their use in the management of constipation.

Phosphorus

Kidney function may decline as senior pets age and CKD is a common cause of poor morbidity and mortality in both dogs and cats. The restriction of dietary phosphorus is a key component in the management of CKD (see Chapter 19), since it can slow progression of the disease (Elliott *et al.*, 2000).

Antioxidants

It has been hypothesized that the ageing process in humans may be associated with an increased oxidative stress state that leads to the release of free radicals (Junqueira *et al.*, 2004). Reactive oxygen species (ROS) is a subset of free radicals, so this umbrella term has been used throughout the chapter. To combat this, antioxidants (e.g. beta-carotene and vitamin E) are often added to senior diets and, theoretically, reduce the speed of ageing as well as support the immune system (Massimo *et al.*, 2003). Although the addition of such antioxidants is unlikely to cause harm, there is currently no evidence to support such benefits. In addition, some antioxidants (e.g. vitamins C and E) may become pro-oxidants if provided in high amounts, although whether this is detrimental remains unclear.

Suitable diet choices

There are many diets available that have been specifically designed for senior pets, but recipes and formulations can differ. Therefore, the choice of diet will depend on the findings of the nutritional assessment and the identification of any risk factors.

Misconceptions about feeding senior pets

Any diet can be fed to a senior pet

Both home-prepared cooked diets (see Chapter 5) and raw meat-based diets (RMBD) (see Chapter 6) pose risks in terms of nutritional adequacy and pathogenic infection. Given that some diet types (e.g. RMBD) use high quantities of phosphorus, they are more likely to deliver unsuitable amounts, which is not desirable when there is concurrent CKD. The risks of pathogenic infection might also be of greater importance in senior pets, whose immune function may be suboptimal. For this reason, RMBDs are not recommended for senior pets, whilst home-prepared cooked diets must be designed and overseen by a suitably qualified person (see Chapter 2).

All senior pets need a lower calorie diet as they are all 'slowing down'

The assumption of lower energy needs in senior pets may not be true in all situations as many seniors remain as active in their adult years, particularly in the earlier senior years (see above). However, when comorbidities affect mobility, energy intake will need to be adjusted so as to avoid unwanted weight gain. Regular weighing and body condition scoring aid in deciding the need to adjust nutritional recommendations to ensure that healthy weight is maintained whilst still meeting all essential nutrient needs.

Communication with pet owners

It is sensible to start conversations with owners early (i.e. prior to the senior years of their pet) about the nutritional changes that may be needed in the future. This will hopefully increase awareness and readiness to change, as well as make owners more receptive to implementing a plan of regular monitoring. Many pet owners will not be aware of the age-related changes to come or may accept clinical signs (e.g. pain) as a normal part of ageing. Tools such as the *BSAVA PetSavers Ageing Canine Toolkit* are a great way to introduce topics for consideration.

Conclusion

Patterns of ageing can vary widely amongst individual dogs and cats. Nutritional recommendations should reflect individual requirements and be based on biological age rather than chronological age and adjusted according to need.

References and further reading

Armstrong PJ (2015) The paradox of healthy obesity. *Purina Companion Animal Nutrition Summit: the future of weight management.* Barcelona, Spain

Bartges JW (2012) Chronic kidney disease in dogs and cats. *Veterinary Clinics of North America: Small Animal Practice* **42(4)**, 669–692

Beale BS (2005) Orthopedic problems in geriatric dogs and cats. *Veterinary Clinics of North America: Small Animal Practice* **35(3)**, 655–674

Bellows J, Colitz CMH, Daristotle L *et al.* (2015) Common physical and functional changes associated with aging in dogs. *Journal of the American Veterinary Medicine Association* **246(1)** 67–75

BSAVA PetSavers (2023) *BSAVA PetSavers Ageing Canine Toolkit.* [Available from: https://bsava.com/petsavers/]

Cave N, Delaney SJ and Larsen JA (2023) Nutritional management of gastrointestinal diseases. In: *Applied Veterinary Clinical Nutrition, 2nd edn.,* ed. AJ Fascetti *et al.,* pp. 235–298. John Wiley & Sons, Inc., Philadelphia

Churchill JA and Eirmann L (2021) Senior pet nutrition and management. *Veterinary Clinics of North America: Small Animal Practice* **51**, 635–651

Cupp CJ, Kerr WW, Jean-Philippe C, Patil AR and Perez-Camargo G (2008) The role of nutritional interventions in the longevity and maintenance of long-term health in aging cats. *International Journal of Applied Research in Veterinary Medicine.* **6(2)**, 69–81

Dhaliwal R, Boynton E, Carrera-Justiz S *et al.* (2023) AAHA senior care guidelines for dogs and cats. *Journal of the American Animal Hospital Association* **59(1)**, 1–21

Donataccio MP, Vanzo A and Bosello O (2021) Obesity paradox and heart failure. *Eating and Weight Disorders* **26**, 1697–1707

Elliott J, Rawlings JM, Markwell PJ and Barber PJ (2000) Survival of cats with naturally occurring chronic renal failure: effect of dietary management. *Journal of Small Animal Practice* **41**, 235–242

Ephraim E, Cochrane CY and Jewell DE (2020) Varying protein levels influence metabolomics and the gut microbiome in healthy adult dogs. *Toxins* **12(8)**, 517

Fascetti A and Delaney S (2012) *Applied Veterinary Clinical Nutrition.* John Wiley & Sons, Ltd., Philadelphia

Fekete SG, Hullár I, Andrásofszky E and Kelemen F (2004) Effect of different fibre types on the digestibility of nutrients in cats. *Journal of Animal Physiology and Animal Nutrition* **88(3–4)**, 138–142

Freeman LM (2018) Cachexia and sarcopenia in companion animals: an underutilized natural animal model of human disease. *JCSM Rapid Communications* **1(2)**, 1–17

Freeman LM, Lachaud MP, Matthews S, Rhodes L and Zollers B (2016) Evaluation of weight loss over time in cats with chronic kidney disease. *Journal of Veterinary Internal Medicine* **30**, 1661–1666

German AJ, Holden SL, Wiseman-Orr ML *et al.* (2012) Quality of life is reduced in obese dogs but improves after successful weight loss. *Veterinary Journal* **192**, 428–434

Gravina G, Ferrari F and Nebbiai G (2021) The obesity paradox and diabetes. *Eating and Weight Disorders* **26**, 1057–1068

Harper EJ (1998) Changing perspectives on aging and energy requirements: aging and energy intake in humans, dogs and cats. *Journal of Nutrition* **128**, S2623–S2626

Junqueira VBC, Barros SBM, Chan SS *et al.* (2004) Aging and oxidative stress. *Molecular Aspects of Medicine* **25(1–2)**, 5–16

Laflamme DP (2005) Nutrition for aging cats and dogs and the importance of body condition. *Veterinary Clinics of North America: Small Animal Practice* **35(3)**, 713–742

Landsberg G and Araujo JA (2005) Behavior problems in geriatric pets. *Veterinary Clinics in North America: Small Animal Practice* **35**, 675–698

Landsberg GM, Deporter T and Araujo JA (2011) Clinical signs and management of anxiety, sleeplessness and cognitive dysfunction in the senior pet. *Veterinary Clinics of North America: Small Animal Practice* **(41)3**, 565–590

Lee DH, Keum N, Hu FB *et al.* (2018) Predicted lean body mass, fat mass, and all cause and cause specific mortality in men: prospective US cohort study. *British Medical Journal* **362**, k2575

Lobprise HB (2017) Dentition and the oral cavity. In: *Treatment and Care of the Geriatric Veterinary Patient,* ed. M Gardner and D McVety, pp. 43–49. John Wiley & Sons, Inc., Philadelphia

Marshall WG, Hazewinkel HAW, Mullen D *et al.* (2010) The effect of weight loss on lameness in obese dogs with osteoarthritis. *Veterinary Research Communication* **34**, 241–253

Martinez-Tapia C, Diot T, Oubaya N *et al.* (2021) The obesity paradox for mid- and long-term mortality in older cancer patients: a prospective multicenter cohort study. *American Journal of Clinical Nutrition* **113**, 129–141

Massimino S, Kearns RJ, Loos KM *et al.* (2003) Effects of age and dietary beta-carotene on immunological variables in dogs. *Journal of Veterinary Internal Medicine* **17**, 835–842

McKenzie BA (2022) Comparative veterinary geroscience: mechanism of molecular, cellular, and tissue aging in humans, laboratory animal models, and companion dogs and cats. *American Journal of Veterinary Research* **(83)6**, doi: 10.2460/ajvr.22.02.0027

Moreno AA, Parker VJ, Winston JA and Rudinsky AJ (2022) Dietary fiber aids in the management of canine and feline gastrointestinal disease. *Journal of the American Veterinary Medical Association* **260(S3)**, S33–S45

O'Neill DG, Church DB, McGreevy PD, Thomson PC and Brodbelt DC (2013) Longevity and mortality of owned dogs in England. *Veterinary Journal* **198**, 638–643

O'Neill DG, Church DB, McGreevy PD, Thomson PC and Brodbelt DC (2015) Longevity and mortality of cats attending primary care veterinary practices in England. *Journal of Feline Medicine and Surgery* **17**, 125–133

Salt C, Morris PJ, Wilson D, Lund EM and German AJ (2018) Association between life span and body condition in neutered client-owned dogs. *Journal of Veterinary Internal Medicine* **33(1)**, 89–99

Salt C, Saito EK, O'Flynn C and Allaway D (2022) Stratification of companion animal life stages from electronic medical record diagnosis data. *The Journals of Gerontology* **78(4)**, 579–586

Slupe JL, Freeman LM and Rush JE (2008) Association of body weight and body condition with survival in dogs with heart failure. *Journal of Veterinary Internal Medicine* **22(3)**, 561–565

Sordo L, Breheny C, Halls V *et al.* (2020) Prevalence of disease and age-related behavioural changes in cats: past and present. *Veterinary Sciences* **7(3)**, 85

Stockman J (2024) Nutrition and aging in dogs and cats. In: *Nutrition and Metabolism of Dogs and Cats*, ed. G Wu, pp. 203–215. Springer Nature, Switzerland

Teng KT, McGreevy PD, Toribio JL, Raubenheimer D, Kendall K and Dhand NK (2018) Strong associations of nine-point body condition scoring with survival and lifespan in cats. *Journal of Feline Medicine and Surgery* **20(12)**, 1110–1118

Woods-Lee G (2023) Senior nutritional requirements for cats and dogs. *Veterinary Nurse* **14**, 393–398

Online extras

This chapter includes:

- A client information leaflet that is available to download and print from the BSAVA Library

Access via QR code or: bsavalibrary.com/nutrition_11

Hospital nutrition

12

'Hospital nutrition' is used to describe nutrition provided within a veterinary hospital. Such nutrition has the potential to directly impact prognosis and speed of recovery. To this end, every attempt should be made to avoid malnutrition in hospitalized patients. Sadly, human hospital studies have shown that 30–50% of patients suffer from malnutrition whilst hospitalized (Konturek *et al.*, 2015); it is thought that a similar problem exists in veterinary hospitals, with 73% of veterinary patients having an energy deficit whilst in the hospital (Remillard *et al.*, 2001). It is vital, therefore, that adequate calories and nutrients be delivered to all hospitalized patients (see Chapter 13 for further information).

Nutritional assessment

All patients need an individualized nutrition plan based on their current health status and the information found during the nutritional assessment. A nutritional assessment should be performed within the first 24 hours or, ideally, at the time that the patient is admitted (see Chapter 2). This assessment should reveal information about the current diet and preferences of the pet, together with any other pertinent information that may affect the hospital nutrition plan, including foods to avoid.

Suitable diet choices

To provide excellent nutrition whilst patients are in the hospital, a wide range of diets should be available, with all diets being complete and balanced for the intended species. In addition, hospitals should stock a range of highly palatable foods that can be used to tempt an anorexic patient to eat. Diet selection will depend on the reason for admission to the hospital and should include:

- Milk replacement formulas
  - For neonates in situations where, for whatever reason, the mother is not available to feed them (see Chapter 10).
- Growth diets
  - Suitable for puppies, kittens or those who may be boarding or brought in as strays (see Chapter 10).
- Maintenance adult diets
  - Suitable for those adult patients who do not have specific nutritional requirements. This may include uncomplicated postoperative patients, boarding patients or those brought in as strays.

- Highly digestible diets
  - Suitable for patients with no additional medical requirement for a specific dietetic food, but who are not consuming food at their usual volume or have a gastrointestinal disturbance. This diet type is typically more energy dense than a maintenance diet, meaning that smaller quantities (compared with a maintenance diet) can be consumed to satisfy energy and nutrient requirements. These diets may also be preferable for hospitalized patients because they allow for ease of digestion with lower residue, resulting in a reduced volume of faecal output.
- Highly digestible, highly palatable diets suitable for growth
- Dietetic food – a range of diets is required and, ideally, should include those suitable for animals with:
  - Renal impairment (i.e. with lower phosphorus concentrations; see Chapter 19)
  - Poor liver function (i.e. with lower copper concentrations and/or alternative protein sources to reduce ammonia accumulation; see Chapter 21)
  - Suspected adverse reactions to food (i.e. hydrolysed or single-protein diets; see Chapter 14)
  - Any condition requiring a low-fat diet.
- Diets suitable for tube feeding (see Chapter 13)
- Single-protein sources (e.g. cooked chicken, ham or tuna); however, these protein sources are to be used to encourage food consumption only and are not to be fed alone.

Feeding plans

Energy requirements and quantities of food should be calculated accurately for all patients and recorded clearly on the hospitalization sheet or on a separate hospital nutritional assessment form (see Chapter 2). Spreadsheets can be devised for this purpose, so all staff members can quickly and accurately calculate feeding quantities (Figure 12.1). Such spreadsheets can then be added to the patient file for review or future reference. The quantities of food offered and consumed should be recorded. All food, be it wet or dry, should be weighed prior to being offered and any remaining food weighed when removed. In this way, actual amounts of food (and therefore calories) consumed can be calculated per day. At the end of each 24-hour period, the quantity of calories consumed should be reviewed and alterations to the nutrition plan made if this amount does not meet the needs of the patient.

Hyporexic and anorexic patients

Time and care should be taken with patients who are hyporexic or anorexic since poor nutrition within the hospital has been associated with negative effects. Factors associated with hyporexia or anorexia include:

- Pain
- Stress
- Disease
- Nausea
- Injury
- Persistent recumbency
- Gastrointestinal obstruction.

Maintenance nutrition plan – canine

Animal's name: Animal's weight (kg): **10**

Clinician: ....   Contact extension:...

BCS: ....   MCS: ....

Current diet: ....

History: ....

....

Daily calorific requirement:	534 Kcal	Food required:	Gastrointestinal
Calorie content in food:	**109 Kcal/100 g**	Total amount of food required:	490 g/day
Day 1	490 g split into	**4** meals = 123 g/meal	

Weigh the patient daily and record on kennel sheets
Always record how much the patient is actually eating to ensure the patient is not hyporexic or anorexic

Figure 12.1: An example of a form for calculating energy requirements and quantities of food. BCS = body condition score; MCS = muscle condition score.
(Courtesy of the University of Liverpool, Small Animal Teaching Hospital)

Elements to consider

To help a patient voluntarily consume the required quantities of food within the hospital, a number of key elements should be considered:

- **Environment**
  - Reduce stress – the environment that each patient is housed in should be evaluated with the aim of reducing stress factors
  - Environmental modifications – modifications should be made (wherever possible) to ensure a quiet, secure place to rest, recover and eat (e.g. moving anorexic patients to quieter areas or providing hiding places for cats; Figure 12.2)
  - Separate resources – cats do not like to eat near their litter tray or their source of water. Food bowls should be placed away from other resources. Larger kennels may be required for cats to facilitate this, and double bowls should be avoided or used for only food or only water, not a mixture of both
  - Change of scenery – taking dogs to a quiet grassy area (not used for toileting) or to a quiet room can encourage them to eat. Since cats are a solitary species, taking them into a quiet consulting room away from other patients for feeding may encourage voluntary food consumption or offering food in the evening when the ward is quieter.

- **Bowl types**
  - For some patients, metal bowls appear to be a deterrent due to their shiny, noisy nature, especially when the patient has to wear an Elizabethan collar which will strike the bowl. Plastic, ceramic or Pyrex® bowls are often tolerated better. However, some patients may have a contact allergy to plastics, so bowl choice should be considered in each individual case

---

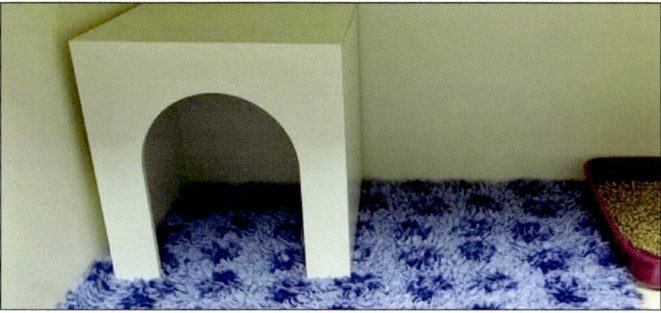

Figure 12.2: Using a hide in the kennel is a good way of reducing stress in cats, especially those that are nervous and like to hide away to feel safe.
(Courtesy of Wood Veterinary Group)

- Cats do not like to get food and water on their whiskers; therefore, wide shallow bowls or saucers or even a tin cover/lid can be used, despite the risk of these being more easily overturned
- For large breeds of dog, those with mobility concerns or with spinal or neck pain who may find eating from a bowl on the floor difficult or even painful, raised bowls may encourage better consumption of food. However, an increased risk of gastric dilatation and volvulus (GDV) has been associated with feeding from raised bowls (Glickman *et al.*, 2000) (see Chapter 18), but in the hospital environment the significance of this remains unclear.

■ **Different foods**
- Only one food type should be offered at any one time
- The patient should be given sufficient time (e.g. 20–30 minutes) to consume the food; if food has not been consumed within this timeframe, then the food should be removed (except in some circumstances, such as cats who prefer to eat at night)
- A new food can then be offered at the next designated time to feed the patient.

■ **Highly palatable foods**
- If the food being offered is refused, a more palatable diet type can be given instead (if suitable for the patient's situation). Foods with a greater moisture, fat and protein content can be more appealing to cats and dogs and might be consumed more readily. A good understanding of the condition of the patient is necessary, because, for example, high fat diets may not be desirable in specific instances, such as in cases of lymphangiectasia
- Highly palatable foods include chicken, ham and tuna. However, since these foods are not complete and balanced if fed alone, they should only be used to encourage the consumption of an optimal complete and balanced diet, rather than being the sole food fed throughout the period of hospitalization.

■ **Positive interactions**
- Hospitalized patients are usually beloved family pets; therefore, allocating time for non-clinical interactions, grooming and affection (if the patient enjoys them) can often encourage them to eat. It is important that more unpleasant interactions, such as temperature taking and injections, are balanced and timed so as not to interfere with interactions the patient might enjoy. This may, to a certain extent, offset the stress and fear some patients will experience in a hospital environment.

- ## Other strategies
  - Removing Elizabethan collars (whilst under constant supervision)
  - Handfeeding (without gloves, if possible)
  - Matching the preferences of the patient – often in hospitals, only wet foods are offered. Cats can be unwilling to depart from their food-type preferences and appear to be neophobic to foods while under stressful conditions (Bradshaw *et al.*, 2000), so dry food should always be offered if the patient usually eats a dry diet at home
  - Warming the food to just below body temperature – this enhances aroma and palatability, which is especially important for any patient with an impaired sense of smell. Cats who cannot smell their food (e.g. in cases of cat influenza) are usually unwilling to consume it, so efforts to maintain their nasal passages, together with warming foods to enhance the smell, can assist in increasing food consumption
  - Providing stronger smelling foods – foods with a pungent aroma, such as oily fish, can encourage consumption
  - Owner presence – having the owner present to tempt the patient to eat, provided they do not become distressed when the owner leaves, and the hospital has a suitable space for this, can be a good strategy to encourage eating
  - Providing favourite foods – owners are often willing to bring in the patient's favourite foods if the hospital does not stock them. Favourite foods may not be complete and balanced and should only be used to encourage the consumption of an appropriate diet. All foods brought in by the pet owner should be cooked; uncooked foods should never be brought into clinical areas of the hospital due to the high pathogen risk these diets present (Freeman *et al.*, 2013) (see Chapter 6).

If the above strategies do not result in the patient consuming sufficient quantities of food, assisted feeding will be required without delay (see Chapter 13).

Other management factors

Learned behaviours and key words

It is useful to ask the pet owner if there are any learned behaviours that have been encouraged at the time of feeding using key words. This may include signals or release words the patient may require before they will eat. This is not only applicable for highly trained service or working dogs, since many pet dogs and cats are asked to wait before being released to eat their food. Failing to gather this information for a patient may delay eating whilst in the hospital.

Misconceptions about hospital nutrition

Chicken alone is suitable to be fed within the hospital

If chicken is fed to a cat or dog as the sole source of food, it will provide only 54% or 62%, respectively, of the essential nutrients required (quantities calculated with the use of an online nutritional formulation tool; BalanceIT). For adult patients, this poses only a small risk, provided the duration of feeding just chicken is limited to only 2–3 days. For patients hospitalized for more than 3 consecutive days, this could pose a significant risk of malnutrition. Therefore, foods consisting of one ingredient (e.g. boiled chicken, canned tuna) should only be used to encourage eating a complete and balanced diet and, wherever possible, not used as the sole food source whilst the patient is under the care of the hospital.

It is best to start a long-term dietetic food within the hospital

In most cases, transition to a diet required for long term feeding, is best performed at home unless a significant dietary alteration is required immediately (e.g. in cases where a low-fat diet is needed). Especially where the diet is pivotal in the management of the patient's condition, transition to a new diet should be carefully controlled and performed over a sufficient amount of time to give the best chance of acceptance (see Chapter 2). In addition, introducing the new diet within the hospital may lead to an association with the negative experience of having an illness and being hospitalized; this is known as an acquired aversion to food and may continue even when the patient returns home (Johnson and Freeman, 2017). For this reason, most food transitions should be initiated when the patient returns home.

Communication with pet owners

For an owner relinquishing their pet to the veterinary team, no matter their level of knowledge or understanding or how much they trust the team, it will be a stressful experience. Time is necessary to discuss all aspects of the pet's stay in the hospital thoroughly and should include information about what the pet will be offered to eat each day. The nutritional assessment upon admission is key to reassuring the owner that all aspects of care have been considered and that their preferences and those of the pet will be taken into account.

When performing a nutritional assessment, veterinary professionals should all be aware that the owner will be in a state of heightened stress and this may affect their ability to recall important information. The pet owner should know who to contact if they remember something important after the appointment. In some cases, for treatment to commence swiftly, the nutritional assessment may be performed by a member of the team other than the veterinary surgeon (veterinarian). Veterinary nurses are well suited to this task, and members of the reception team can also gather basic information, for example about what the pet would usually eat at home and their food and feeding management preferences.

In addition, owners may benefit from a brief description, either verbal or written, of what they can expect their pet to eat while in the hospital. Information can be prepared to be delivered with the other paperwork handed over to the owner upon admittance of the patient. This also affords an opportunity to divulge the practice's policy on the feeding of non-standard diets (e.g. raw diets) within the hospital and describe the alternatives that will be used.

Conclusion

Feeding patients within the hospital can be challenging. With many different conditions and preferences to manage, finding foods that patients want to consume whilst delivering excellent nutrition and preventing malnutrition can prove difficult. With a thorough nutritional assessment, a wide range of diets and foods, and careful thought about the requirements of each individual patient, an excellent standard of nutrition can be provided for all hospitalized cats and dogs.

References and further reading

Bradshaw JWS, Healey LM, Thorne CJ, MacDonald DW and Arden-Clark C (2000) Differences in food preferences between individuals and populations of domestic cats *Felis silvestris catus. Applied Animal Behaviour Science* **68**, 257–268

Freeman LM, Chandler ML, Hamper BA and Weeth LP (2013) Current knowledge about the risks and benefits of raw meat-based diets for dogs and cats. *Journal of the American Veterinary Medical Association* **243**, 1549–1558

Glickman LT, Glickman NW, Schellenberg DB, Raghavan M and Lee T (2000) Non-dietary risk factors for gastric dilatation volvulus in large and giant breed dogs. *Journal of the American Veterinary Medical Association* **217**, 1492–1499

Johnson LN and Freeman LM (2017) Recognizing, describing, and managing reduced food intake in dogs and cats. *Journal of the American Veterinary Medical Association* **251**, 1260–1266

Konturek PC, Herrmann HJ, Schink K, Neurath MF and Zopf Y (2015) Malnutrition in hospitals: it was, is now, and must not remain a problem! *Medical Science Monitor* **21**, 2969–2975

National Research Council (2006) *Nutrient Requirements of Dogs and Cats.* National Academies Press, Washington DC

Remillard RL, Darden DE, Michel KE *et al.* (2001) An investigation of the relationship between caloric intake and outcome in hospitalized dogs. *Veterinary Therapeutics* **2**, 301–310

Useful websites

BalanceIT
https://balance.it/

Online extras

This chapter includes:

- **A client information leaflet that is available to download and print from the BSAVA Library**

Access via QR code or: bsavalibrary.com/nutrition_12

Critical care nutrition

13

Critical care nutrition is provided to those patients within veterinary hospitals who require close monitoring and nursing care or those who are unwilling or unable to consume sufficient food voluntarily due to illness or injury. Provision of nutrition to patients within the veterinary hospital has the potential to impact the outcome of treatment significantly. To promote a timely return of the patient to the owner, malnutrition within the veterinary hospital should be avoided (see Chapter 12). Nutrient and energy deficits directly decrease the ability of the patient to recover. Poor nutrition leads to prolonged healing times, impaired immunity, altered metabolism of drugs and extended periods of hospitalization, all of which are of particular concern for the most vulnerable critical patients (Saker and Remillard, 2010).

Nutritional deficiencies and the associated concerns are not limited to long-term critical patients alone – even in the short term, malnutrition should be avoided because metabolic alterations can be observed after just 3 days of hyporexia or anorexia due to insufficient energy and nutrients (Chan, 2004). This includes the time the patient may not have been eating prior to hospital admission, as well as any periods of hyporexia or anorexia within the hospital. When determining whether to intervene, it is essential to have a clear understanding of when the patient last ate, what was eaten and how much.

Provided that the animal is haemodynamically stable and properly hydrated, a timely nutrition plan should be instigated. This approach is relevant to all patients, including those that are critically ill, with nutrition delivered by a means appropriate for the individual. The nutrition plan should be accurately formulated and instructions clearly communicated to all veterinary hospital staff caring for the patient (see Chapter 2). The nutrition plan should be followed alongside all other medical management and hospitalization instructions. A bespoke form for critical care nutrition should be used so that the complex nutritional plans that are usually needed, can be appropriately designed and executed. Compliance with the plan should be recorded on the form throughout the period of hospitalization, and performance reviewed regularly to ensure that nutritional requirements are being met.

Food reintroduction

Following a period of hyporexia or anorexia, food should be gradually reintroduced to prevent refeeding syndrome, which is rare but can cause serious complications as a result of electrolyte disturbances such as hypophosphataemia. A staged approach to food reintroduction (over 3–4 days) is therefore recommended. The timeframe in which food is reintroduced can vary and more gradual increases are sometimes needed. The response of the patient should be assessed daily to ensure that they are tolerating the feeding before the next increment is made.

Assisted feeding

When a patient will not eat voluntarily, despite efforts to tempt them (see Chapter 12), assisted feeding should be introduced. Methods of assisted feeding include:

- **Medication**
  - Appetite stimulants should be used alongside all efforts to tempt the patient to voluntarily consume foods they are likely to find appetizing
  - Mirtazapine can be given to both cats and dogs, but typically have only a minimal effect on encouraging voluntary food consumption. Dosages can be found in the *BSAVA Small Animal Formulary*
  - Antiemetics may be helpful (e.g. maropitant) where nausea is a primary reason for inappetence
  - Capromorelin (Entyce®), a ghrelin receptor agonist, has recently become licensed in North America and has been shown to be an effective appetite stimulant in dogs (Rhodes *et al.*, 2018). Availability in other countries is more limited; for example, an import licence is required in the UK.
- **Syringe feeding**
  - Force-feeding a patient by delivering liquid food orally using a syringe, should be avoided. It is unpleasant and stressful for the patient and may cause resentment of being handled. In contrast, gently introducing food into the cheek pouch or on to the tongue of a patient with a syringe may encourage eating, especially in cats. However, it is unlikely that this method of feeding will meet energy requirements, so other assisted feeding techniques should be utilized in most circumstances
  - For neonates, gentle syringe feeding may be appropriate; however, care must be taken not to flood the airway with food to prevent aspiration pneumonia (see Chapter 10).
- **Feeding tubes**
  - Feeding tubes are used to deliver sufficient nutrition to a patient in the absence of voluntary food consumption and are often the most appropriate means of providing nutritional support (Figure 13.1). Wrongly considered to be a method of last resort, it is preferable to consider tube feeding sooner rather than later. Cases where tube feeding may be necessary include upper gastrointestinal tract disorders (e.g. oesophageal disease), disorders affecting deglutition (e.g. fractured jaw), alimentary organ diseases (e.g. pancreatic disease, liver disease) and systemic diseases associated with hyporexia or anorexia (e.g. renal disease). Wherever possible, the gastrointestinal tract should be utilized for nutrient and energy absorption
  - Feeding tube selection will depend on the disease status of the patient, the duration assisted feeding is likely to be required for and the availability of equipment and surgical (or other) expertise to place each tube type
  - For neonates, feeding tubes can be an easier and safer option than syringe feeding as it reduces the risk of aspiration pneumonia.

Parenteral nutrition

Parenteral nutrition is that which is administered elsewhere in the body other than the mouth and alimentary canal. This approach is not commonly used in veterinary practice. It is required in rare cases, for example when the entire gastrointestinal tract is not available, or there is malabsorption. Total nutritional support can be delivered via an intravenous catheter placed in the jugular vein or vena cava via the saphenous vein (Figure 13.5). Peripheral parenteral nutrition (PPN) can only provide partial nutritional support because

Feeding tube	Advantages	Disadvantages
Naso-oesophageal or nasogastric tubes		
■ Placed via the nares (Figure 13.2) ■ Duration of use: 3–10 days ■ Tube diameter: 5–8 Fr	■ Can be placed without a general anaesthetic ■ Low risk of infection as naso-oesophageal and nasogastric tubes do not have an associated stoma at the point of entry into the patient's body ■ Minimal equipment required ■ Can be placed rapidly	■ Short-term use only ■ Must be secured with glue or sutures to the head or face, which may become dislodged ■ Once placed and secured, the tube can be dislodged by sneezing or patient interference ■ Tube displacement may cause subsequent aspiration of food ■ Elizabethan collars must be worn to prevent patient interference. Collars are not always well tolerated and may hinder the patient's attempts to consume food voluntarily should their appetite improve ■ Only tubes with a very small diameter can be used (size is restricted by the diameter of the nares). Suitable diets for the patient's condition may not be available in an appropriate consistency to pass down such narrow tubes. A large volume of water may have to be added to make suitable diets liquid enough to pass down the tube. Large volumes may not be desirable
Oesophagostomy tubes		
■ Surgically placed into the oesophagus via the lateral neck (Figure 13.3)	■ Mid-term use ■ Straightforward to place and tolerated well in most cases with limited patient interference	■ Requires a short general anaesthetic to place. The patient must be haemodynamically stable and well enough to withstand an anaesthetic

Figure 13.1: Types of feeding tube that can be used to provide nutritional support. (continues) ▶

Feeding tube	Advantages	Disadvantages
Oesophagostomy tubes (continues)		
■ Duration of use: weeks to months ■ Tube diameter: 8–19 Fr ■ For details on the care and safe use of oesophagostomy tubes, see text	■ Wider bore than naso-oesophageal or nasogastric tubes, allowing suitable foods to be administered more easily, although dilution of canned diets may still be required ■ An Elizabethan collar is not required in most cases ■ Food can be offered for voluntary consumption, provided no functional restriction is present that would prevent it ■ Suitable for at-home use by a pet owner after a demonstration has been given. This allows for a shorter duration of hospitalization	■ Risk of stoma site infection. The stoma should be cleaned using an aseptic technique and fresh dressings applied daily ■ Can be dislodged by vomiting ■ Can become blocked if proper flushing is not undertaken prior to feeding ■ Risk of tube displacement and subsequent aspiration of food
Gastrostomy tubes		
■ Placed percutaneously, endoscopically or surgically (Figure 13.4) ■ Duration of use: >6 months ■ Tube diameter: 16–28 Fr	■ Long-term assisted feeding ■ Wide-bore tubes that allow suitable diets to be administered with minimal preparation ■ Tolerated well in most cases ■ Likelihood of patient interference is low ■ No need for an Elizabethan collar in most cases ■ Food can be offered for voluntary consumption ■ Intended for use at home by the pet owner	■ Requires a general anaesthetic to place ■ Specialist equipment (e.g. an endoscope) and skilled staff are required ■ Risk of stoma site infection

Figure 13.1: (continued) Types of feeding tube that can be used to provide nutritional support.

of the osmolality of the solution needed. This form of nutrition can be a good adjunct to partial enteral feeding when a patient cannot cope with 100% of the resting energy requirement (RER) being administered enterally.

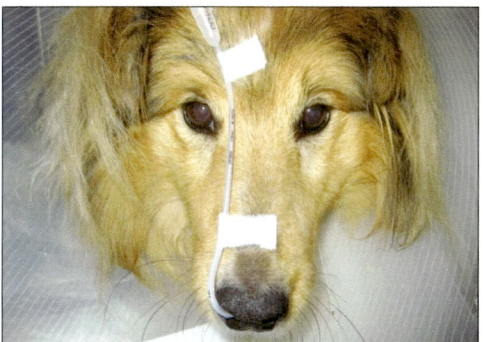

Figure 13.2: Dog with a naso-oesophageal feeding tube in place that has been secured with tape and glue (sutures can also be used).
(Reproduced from the *BSAVA Textbook of Veterinary Nursing*)

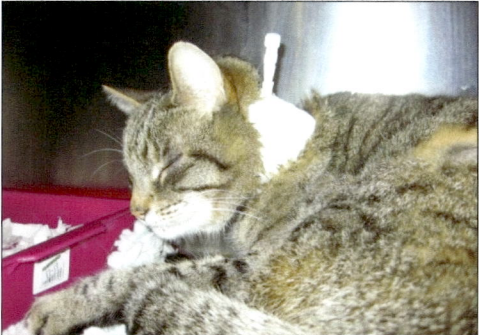

Figure 13.3: A cat with an oesophagostomy feeding tube in place.
(Reproduced from the *BSAVA Textbook of Veterinary Nursing*)

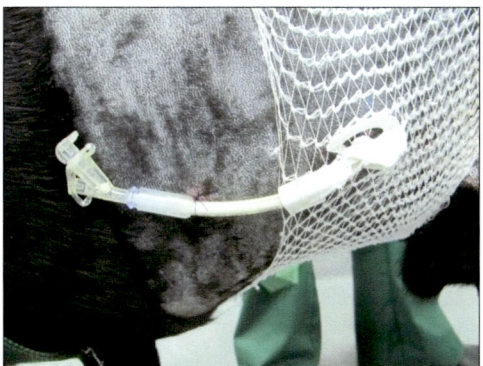

Figure 13.4: A percutaneous endoscopic gastrostomy (PEG) tube secured in a dog using a body stockinet.
(Reproduced from the *BSAVA Textbook of Veterinary Nursing*)

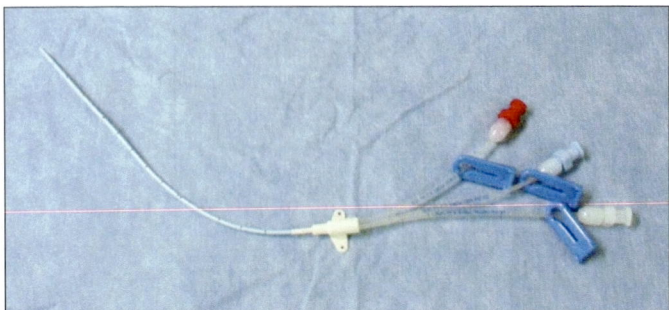

Figure 13.5: Parenteral nutrition is best administered via dedicated catheters designed for long-term use. A triple lumen central catheter is commonly used.
(Reproduced from the *BSAVA Manual of Canine and Feline Advanced Veterinary Nursing*)

Calculating feeding requirements

Step 1: Calculate total energy requirements

The most appropriate calculation for critical patients is the RER, which can be calculated as follows:

- For patients weighing 2–30 kg:
  - (bodyweight x 30) + 70 = RER (kcal/day)
- For all patients (including those weighing <2 kg or >30 kg):
  - 70 x bodyweight $^{0.75}$ = RER (kcal/day)

Step 2: Decide on the most appropriate food

Food choice will be based on the requirements of the individual patient and the availability of suitable liquid diets or food blenders that can bring diets to a suitable consistency for feeding tubes (see below).

Step 3: Determine calorie content and calculate the necessary quantity of food

The caloric content of the chosen diet should be determined for 100 g of food. This information can be acquired by calculating it from the analytical constituents on the packaging (see Chapter 2), by reading any associated literature from the food manufacturer (e.g. product books) or by contacting the manufacturer. Once the caloric content is known, the following calculation will be necessary to determine feeding quantities:

- (RER / calories in 100 g of food) x 100 = amount of food to feed per 24 hours (g)

Step 4: Determine the quantity of food to be given per day, if different from the full RER

This is known as the daily energy requirement (DER). Should a staged reintroduction of food be required, the calorie quantity should be reintroduced slowly over 3-4 days (depending on the duration of the hyporexia or anorexia). An example of a 3-day reintroduction of food is as follows:

- DER day 1 = 1/3 of RER
- DER day 2 = 2/3 of RER
- DER day 3 = full RER.

Step 5: Determine the quantity of food to be given per meal

When using feeding tubes, smaller, more frequent meals are desired to reduce the risk of vomiting; therefore, the total daily food quantity should be divided into four or more meals.

Example

Feeding quantity calculation for a critical patient who has a feeding tube and requires a staged reintroduction of food:

- **Patient details:** Domestic Shorthaired cat; male; neutered; 8 years old; bodyweight = 4.5 kg; body condition score (BCS) = 5/9; muscle condition score (MCS) = normal
- **Current diet:** Commercially produced wet and dry diet
- **Reason for hospitalization:** Fractured jaw following a road traffic accident; anorexic for 3–4 days
- **Energy requirement:**
  - RER = (4.5 × 30) + 70 = 205 kcal/day
- **Chosen food:** High-energy, nutrient-dense, wet food preparation (note: there are many food options available in this category)
- **Calorie content of food:** 120 kcal/100 g
- **Feeding amount required:** (205/120) x 100 = 171 g per day (full RER amount)
- **Staged reintroduction of food:**
  - Day 1 (1/3 RER) = 171/3 = 57 g
  - Day 2 (2/3 RER) = (171/3) x 2 = 114 g
  - Day 3 and thereafter (full RER) = 171 g

Given that feeding calculations can be complex and time-consuming, designing spreadsheets to calculate feeding amounts rapidly and accurately minimizes the chance of errors (Figure 13.6). Such documents can be saved to the patient's file to provide a record of the feeding plan, as well as how quantities were determined. A list of the calorie content of commonly stocked foods is very helpful to use alongside these spreadsheets, or to have on file, thus reducing the need for recalculation for each new patient that requires a tube feeding plan.

Suitable diet choices

Pre-prepared liquid formulations specifically designed for use with feeding tubes are readily available for different medical conditions. However, especially for large breeds of dog, this can become an expensive method of feeding. Alternatively, dietetic or other food can be blended with water in a food processor to become a slurry thin enough to be delivered via a feeding tube. The added water must be accounted for in all feeding quantity calculations. The disadvantages of blending dietetic food include the difficulty of obtaining an optimal consistency for very narrow-bore tubes without using a large amount of water, which would then greatly increase the volume of food delivered to the patient and decrease the caloric density. This may be contraindicated in the presence of delayed

---

ICU/feeding tubes nutrition plan – canine	
Animal's name:	Animal's weight (kg): **10**
Clinician:	Contact extension: ....
BCS:	MCS: ....
Current diet:	
History:	

Daily calorific requirement: 370 Kcal	Food required:	
Calorie content in food: **391 Kcal/100 g**	Total amount of food required: 95 g/day	

If using PEG or oesophagostomy tubes, see separate sheets for instructions on how to feed. Please split the meals as below, the total requirement should be gradually increased over 3 days to reach total amount on day 3 (48 hours after starting to feed).

Day 1 (1/3 total amount)	32 g split into	**5** meals =	6 g/meal
Day 2 (2/3 total amount)	63 g split into	**5** meals =	13 g/meal
Day 3 (full amount)	95 g split into	**5** meals =	19 g/meal

If no assisted feeding is required, start on full amount on day 1

Day 1	95 g split into	**5** meals =	19 g/meal

Weigh the patient daily and record on kennel sheets
Always record how much the patient is actually eating to ensure not hyporexic or anorexic

Figure 13.6: An example of a form for calculating energy requirements and quantities of food for assisted feeding. BCS = body condition score; MCS = muscle condition score; PEG = percutaneous endoscopic gastrotomy.
(Courtesy of the University of Liverpool, Small Animal Teaching Hospital)

gastric emptying or may cause the patient to vomit. Very large feed volumes can be delivered via constant rate infusions, provided the necessary equipment and monitoring are available. For excitable patients, this may not be a suitable option.

Other management factors

Care and safe use of oesophageal feeding tubes

Insertion site inspection
Inspection of the insertion site should be undertaken on a daily basis. Personal protective equipment (PPE), such as gloves, is required to minimize the risk of introducing infection to the stoma site.

1. Remove bandages and dressings from around the tube.
2. Inspect the stoma site for infection.
3. Gently clean around the tube at the insertion site.
4. Dry the area.
5. Reapply a fresh dressing and bandage.

Feeding by bolus
During preparation for tube feeding, highly palatable food should always be offered for voluntary consumption, if oral intake is appropriate for the patient. Should the patient voluntarily consume food that is equivalent to >80% of the required amount, tube feeding may not be required. However, should the patient not consume food in a similar manner at the next meal, tube feeding will still be necessary.

1. Prepare all equipment needed:
   a. 1 x empty 5 ml syringe
   b. 1 × 5 ml syringe for sterile water
   c. 1 × 5 ml syringe for tap water
   d. Appropriately sized syringes for the selected food; 60 ml syringes are a good option for large feeding volumes.
2. Ensure food and liquids are at the correct temperature for administration:
   a. Sterile water and tap water should be at room temperature (warmed if necessary); the administration of hot and/or cold fluids should be avoided
   b. Food should be at body temperature. Syringes should be capped to prevent leakage of food contents and then placed in a warm water bath until the desired temperature is reached. Syringes should never be heated in a microwave as this creates hotspots or melts them.
3. Check whether any medication is to be given with the food; prepare if required. This may involve crushing some medications to be delivered via the tube along with the food.
4. Confirm correct tube position:
   a. Clean the delivery port
   b. Uncap the tube, but keep the tubing pinched and occluded until a syringe is attached
   c. Attach the empty syringe and draw back. Negative pressure should be observed on drawback
      i. Should air enter the syringe freely, the tube may have become dislodged and could now be in the airway
      ii. Should stomach contents appear in the syringe, insufficient time has elapsed since the last feed, the stomach may not be emptying correctly, or vomiting has occurred
      iii. In both cases, the veterinary team should review the situation and decide how to proceed.
   d. Pinch and occlude the tube whilst changing the empty syringe for the one containing sterile water
   e. Flush the tube with 2–5 ml of sterile water and monitor for a cough. Stop introducing water immediately if a cough is observed; however, the absence of a cough does not guarantee that the tube has not been displaced to the airway.
5. Deliver the full food quantity:
   a. Once correct tube position has been confirmed, commence delivery of the food
   b. Pinch and occlude the tube whilst replacing the syringe that contained sterile water for the one containing food
   c. Delivery of the food volume should be slow, taking 5–20 minutes (depending on the size of the patient, its response and the volume to be given). If salivation or gulping is observed, slow the rate of infusion by 50% and observe further throughout a slower delivery. Too rapid an introduction of food can cause vomiting. In this case, the delivery of food should be slowed to 1 ml/minute if no other cause is suspected
   d. Take the opportunity to give the patient some positive attention (e.g. grooming) whilst feeding. This may help to make tube feeding a pleasant experience and so reduce the risk of the patient resenting the process.
6. Complete the final steps:
   a. Once the feed has been completed, pinch and occlude the tube whilst changing the now empty food syringe for the 5 ml syringe containing tap water. Sterile water is not necessary for this process as correct tube position has already been confirmed

b. Flush the tube to clear it of any remaining food or medications
c. Ensure all dressings remain clean and dry – replace them if needed
d. Cap the feeding tube and tuck it out of the way to prevent it from catching and becoming dislodged or annoying the patient. The use of stockinet dressings over the neck dressing can be very useful for this purpose. Specific oesophagostomy tube neck collars are also available
e. Make sure the patient is clean and dry (cats, especially, are fastidious cleaners of their coat).

As voluntary consumption resumes, provided the patient is consuming enough food to maintain their bodyweight, the feeding tube can be removed.

Misconceptions about critical care nutrition

Carbonated drinks can be used to unblock feeding tubes

Carbonated drinks may assist with unblocking feeding tubes if they have become occluded. However, the use of high-sugar drinks, which may significantly increase the blood glucose concentration of the patient if given in large quantities, is rarely desirable and caution should be exercised. Carbonated drinks may also contain phosphoric acid, which is undesirable for some patients. Moreover, water alone has been found to be more effective than any carbonated drink or cranberry juice for unblocking feeding tubes. The best solution to dissolve such occlusions has been found to be 325 mg of sodium bicarbonate and a quarter of a teaspoon of pancreatic enzyme mixed together in 5 ml of water (Parker and Freeman, 2013). Diligent prevention of blockages by sufficiently flushing the feeding tube after all feeds is strongly recommended.

Weight loss is inevitable in critical patients with feeding tubes

Provided sufficient energy is delivered, bodyweight can be maintained via all types of feeding tubes in many patients. However, for patients in a catabolic state, weight loss is inevitable despite the use of a feeding tube. In addition, determining the exact energy requirements for each individual is not possible, so monitoring is key, and patients should be weighed daily to ensure their weight remains stable. During the initial few days when food reintroduction is taking place, a slight weight loss may be observed; however, this should not continue once the full DER is being delivered.

Conclusion

Critically ill patients require significant veterinary treatment and care, and the provision of nutrition is vital for a good recovery and a timely return home to the pet owner. Even if voluntary intake is absent, there are many suitable options to continue to provide nutrition and every critical patient should have an individualized, detailed nutrition plan created and implemented as soon as it is feasible to do so.

References and further reading

Allerton F (2023) *BSAVA Small Animal Formulary, 11th edition – Part A: Canine and Feline*. BSAVA Publications, Gloucester

Chan DL (2004) Nutritional requirements of the critically ill patient. *Clinical Techniques in Small Animal Practice* **19**, 1–5

Cooper B, Mullineaux E and Turner L (2020) *BSAVA Textbook of Veterinary Nursing, 6th edn*. BSAVA Publications, Gloucester

Konturek PC, Herrmann HJ, Schink K, Neurath MF and Zopf Y (2015) Malnutrition in hospitals: it was, is now, and must not remain a problem! *Medical Science Monitor* **21**, 2969–2975

Moore AH and Rudd S (2008) *BSAVA Manual of Canine and Feline Advanced Veterinary Nursing, 2nd edn*. BSAVA Publications, Gloucester

Parker VJ and Freeman LM (2013) Comparison of various solutions to dissolve critical care diet clots. *Journal of Veterinary Emergency and Critical Care* **23**, 344–347

Remillard RL, Darden DE, Michel KE *et al.* (2001) An investigation of the relationship between caloric intake and outcome in hospitalized dogs. *Veterinary Therapeutics* **2**, 301–310

Rhodes L, Zollers B, Wofford JA and Heinen E (2018) Capromorelin: a ghrelin receptor agonist and novel therapy for stimulation of appetite in dogs. *Veterinary Medicine and Science* **4**, 3–16

Saker KE and Remillard RL (2010) Critical care nutrition and enteral-assisted feeding. In: *Small Animal Clinical Nutrition, 5th edn*, ed. MS Hand *et al.*, pp. 439–476. Mark Morris Institute, Topeka

Online extras

This chapter includes:

● **A client information leaflet that is available to download and print from the BSAVA Library**

Access via QR code or: bsavalibrary.com/nutrition_13

Adverse reactions to food

14

When animals suffer an adverse reaction to food, correct identification of the cause(s) of the reaction is key to providing an effective nutritional management strategy. Veterinary professionals need to provide guidance about identification of the source of the reaction, as well as about suitable diets that meet the requirements of the patient. An adverse reaction to food may be due to:

- Dietary indiscretion
- Food intolerance
- Food poisoning
- Food allergy (hypersensitivity).

Genuine adverse food reactions account for only 1% of skin disease cases seen in practice, making it uncommon (Case *et al.*, 2000). Food-associated gastrointestinal disease is common in cats and dogs, but only a minority of cases have been proven to be the result of a genuine immune-mediated food hypersensitivity (i.e. allergy; Olivry and Mueller, 2019). Instead, most arise through other pathogenetic mechanisms (e.g. intolerances). For these reasons the term 'adverse food reaction' is preferred to 'food allergy'.

Clinically, adverse food reactions most often manifest with gastrointestinal or dermatological signs or both (Figure 14.1). In the USA, studies found that the following ingredients were associated with a cutaneous adverse reaction (Roudebush *et al.*, 2010):

- In dogs:
  - Beef
  - Dairy products
  - Soya
  - Wheat.
- In cats:
  - Beef
  - Dairy products
  - Fish.

These associations largely reflect ingredients that are commonly included in diets and, as a result, they are likely to vary between countries and pet populations.

The effect of nutrition

Given that certain ingredients within a fed diet are responsible for adverse reactions, altering the diet is the best way both of determining the cause and of preventing further

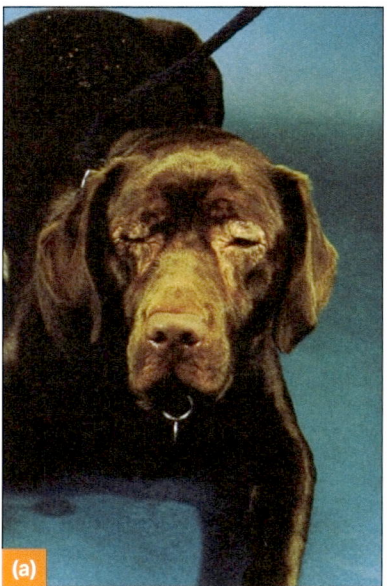
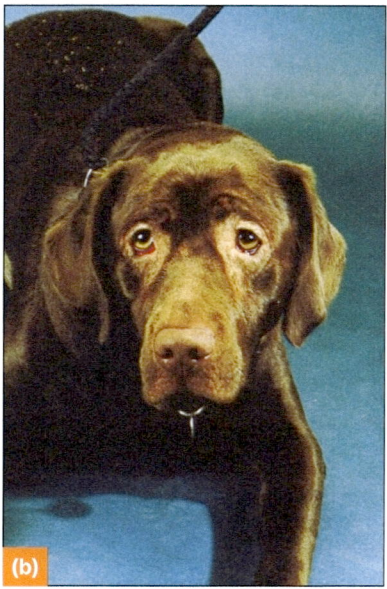

Figure 14.1: (a) A 10-month-old neutered Labrador Retriever bitch with a food-responsive dermatosis. The clinical signs are concentrated on the face. (b) The same dog after 4 weeks on a hypoallergenic diet trial.
(Reproduced from the *BSAVA Manual of Canine and Feline Dermatology*)

reactions long term. If possible, this should be undertaken in a formal food elimination trial (Case *et al.*, 2000). Although serology and saliva testing for food allergens are comercially available, they are unreliable and, therefore, should not be used (Jeffers *et al.*, 1991).

Conducting a food elimination trial

Step 1: Conduct a nutritional review

The dietary history should be thoroughly reviewed and used to create a list of ingredients within the animal's diet including those in the main meal and extras (e.g. treats, food scraps, supplements and foods used to administer medications). Recording details of the medications administered is also recommended because these can sometimes contain nutritional components (especially 'chewable' preparations and medicines in capsules typically synthesized from bovine or porcine gelatine).

Step 2: Select an appropriate diet

Appropriate diets are typically one of the following:

- **Novel** – a diet comprising a single carbohydrate and protein source that the pet has not consumed in the past
- **Hydrolysed** – a diet formulated from a modified protein source, by chemical or enzymatic means, to reduce its molecular size, typically to a concentration below 10,000 Daltons (Roudebush *et al.*, 2010). It is claimed that at this size, the protein molecules are less likely to cause a hypersensitivity reaction.

113

Step 3: Exclusively feed the chosen diet

The necessity for complete compliance with feeding the selected diet should be stressed to the owner, as feeding additional foods may render the results of the trial inconclusive. Ideally, the administration of medication should also be avoided during the trial as some formulations may contain nutritional components (see above).

Step 4: Decide upon a feeding duration

For those with gastrointestinal reactions, the initial elimination phase should last for 2 weeks, which is usually sufficient time as clinical signs typically resolve in 7–10 days. For patients with dermatological signs, the trial period should last for 6–10 weeks (Rosser, 1993). A positive response occurs when the clinical signs have diminished by the end of the trial period. Should the clinical signs remain, this could indicate another cause (e.g. a disease that is not of dietary origin), a possible reaction to one of the ingredients chosen for the trial or insufficient time on the trial diet. Some patients (particularly those with dermatological signs) may require a trial period of more than 12 weeks, whereas others will respond in just 3 weeks. Some patients may require a trial with other diets if they do not respond to the first diet trial.

Step 5: Re-challenge for the first time

Once the pet has completed the initial elimination phase, they should be re-challenged with their original diet to determine whether there is a relapse of clinical signs. A return of signs within 2 weeks is indicative of a reaction to one or more of the ingredients within the original food (Jeffers *et al.*, 1991). The identification of specific ingredients is now required. However, many pet owners will be unwilling to re-challenge their pet (or undertake secondary re-challenge) for fear of the clinical signs returning. In such cases, feeding the trial diet long term can be considered; this can be undertaken, provided that the trial diet is complete and balanced for all essential nutrients.

Step 6: Return to the trial diet

The pet should now be returned to the trial diet, and it should be fed until the clinical signs subside once again.

Step 7: Re-challenge for the second time

The pet should now be reintroduced to one food ingredient at a time and carefully monitored for any reactions. If no reaction is observed, another ingredient may be introduced. The return of clinical signs would indicate a reaction to the ingredient of concern. This ingredient should be withdrawn and the process of rechallenge continued systematically until all common ingredients have been tested.

Suitable diet choices

A suitable diet for a pet with an adverse reaction to food is one that does not contain ingredients that they are known to react to (ideally identified during a food elimination trial). This may be a novel maintenance diet, a dietetic food or, where no commercially produced diet is suitable, a home-prepared cooked diet (see Chapter 5). In this case, it is recommended that the recipe be designed, overseen or approved by an individual with appropriate qualifications (see Chapter 2).

Misconceptions about adverse reactions to food

Owners can still give treats during the diet trial

Owners are likely to give treats as part of their normal interactions with their pet, so they should be advised to use part of the daily allocation of the elimination diet as treats throughout the trial period. Any foods other than the trial diet must not be fed or they will invalidate the trial and the results will not identify which food ingredients are causing a reaction.

Feeding a grain-free diet will prevent 'food allergies'

A strict grain-free diet is only necessary for those pets who have a proven reaction to grains (e.g. in cases of gluten-sensitive dyskinesia; Lowrie *et al.*, 2015). There is no evidence that feeding diets containing grains causes adverse reactions to food and, therefore, feeding a grain-free diet is unlikely to prevent them. Recent research has highlighted significant concerns with the feeding of some grain-free diets and the development of cardiomyopathy in dogs, although exact mechanisms are unclear. However, it is more likely to be associated with the inclusion of other ingredients (e.g. some pulses) in the diet. Therefore, except for dogs and cats proven to react adversely to grains, it is not necessary to feed a grain-free diet.

Homemade diets are the best choice for a pet with 'food allergies'

If the home-prepared cooked diet is formulated and overseen by an individual with a suitable qualification (see above) who ensures that the diet is complete and balanced, it is certainly a suitable option; however, there are many potential pitfalls associated with feeding homemade diets. The majority have been found to be nutritionally inadequate (Heinze *et al.*, 2012; Larsen *et al.*, 2012; Stockman *et al.*, 2013), especially when recipes from the internet, books or magazines are used or when expert guidance has not been sought. Furthermore, even if the recipe has been correctly formulated, it still relies upon the pet owner following the recipe precisely and consistently (see Chapter 5).

Preventing recurrence of an adverse reaction to food

Depending on the underlying cause, further reactions should be prevented by good compliance with the dietary recommendation and/or by prevention of dietary indiscretions through environmental changes (e.g. securing the lid of the waste bin so it can not be accessed).

Communication with pet owners

A diagnosis of an adverse reaction to food may be readily accepted by some owners, for example when there is only one pet within the household, when the source of a single ingredient can easily be eliminated from the diet or when a simple environmental alteration can be used to prevent access. When multiple ingredients are responsible for the adverse reaction, strict compliance can be more difficult for an owner to maintain. A holistic view should be taken, which includes the pet, owner and home environment. Owners need to be made aware of the wider implications of the recommendation. Wider implications may include the diet chosen for other pets, ingredients in purchased treats and any scraps of food which the pet may regularly receive from the owner. To maintain compliance with the restriction of specific ingredients of concern, removal of the ingredient from the entire household may be required, particularly if the pet regularly steals food. Challenges with implementing any recommendations should be discussed, and ongoing owner support may be required. If food sharing between pets in the household is a frequent occurrence, owners will need to develop strategies to minimize or eliminate this altogether; although, provided that the new food is complete and balanced, it should not present any problems for the other, unaffected healthy pet(s). In a multi-pet household, a successful plan might require the diet of all pets to be changed to avoid any risk of exposure. Another solution for cats and small dogs fed dry diets is to use a microchip-activated food bowl, meaning only the designated pet can consume the food within it. It may be necessary to segregate larger dogs during feeding.

Conclusion

Adverse reactions to food can occur for several reasons; effective management relies upon identification of the source of the reaction and subsequent elimination of the ingredients of concern. Provision of optimal nutrition with good dietary compliance is central to successful management and maintenance of good health in these cases.

References and further reading

Case LP, Carey DP, Hirakawa DA and Daristotle L (2000) *Canine and Feline Nutrition.* Mosby, Maryland Heights

Heinze CR, Gomez FC and Freeman LM (2012) Assessment of commercial diets and recipes for home-prepared diets recommended for dogs with cancer. *Journal of the American Veterinary Medical Association* **241**, 1453–1460

Jackson HA and Marsella R (2012) *BSAVA Manual of Canine and Feline Dermatology, 3rd edn.* BSAVA Publications, Gloucester

Jeffers JG, Shanley KJ and Meyer EK (1991) Diagnostic testing of dogs for food hypersensitivity. *Journal of the American Veterinary Medical Association* **198**, 245–250

Larsen JA, Parks EM, Heinze CR and Fascetti AJ (2012) Evaluation of recipes for home-prepared diets for dogs and cats with chronic kidney disease. *Journal of the American Veterinary Medical Association* **240**, 532–538

Lowrie M, Garden OA, Hadjivassiliou M *et al.* (2015) The clinical and serological effect of a gluten-free diet in Border Terriers with epileptoid cramping syndrome. *Journal of Veterinary Internal Medicine* **29**, 1564–1568

Olivry T and Mueller RS (2019) Critically appraised topic on adverse food reactions (7): signalment and cutaneous manifestations of dogs and cats with adverse food reactions. *BMC Veterinary Research* **15**, 140

Rosser EJ (1993) Diagnosis of food allergy in dogs. *Journal of the American Veterinary Medical Association* **203**, 259–262

Roudebush P, Guilford WG and Jackson HA (2010) Adverse reactions to food. In: *Small Animal Clinical Nutrition, 5th edn*, ed. MS Hand *et al.*, pp. 609–634. Mark Morris Institute, Topeka

Stockman J, Fascetti AJ, Kass PH and Larsen JA (2013) Evaluation of recipes of home-prepared maintenance diets for dogs. *Journal of the American Veterinary Medical Association* **242**, 1500–1505

Online extras

This chapter includes:

- A client information leaflet that is available to download and print from the BSAVA Library

Access via QR code or: bsavalibrary.com/nutrition_14

Obesity care

15

The field of canine and feline nutrition is vast with an ever changing and evolving landscape, not least when it comes to obesity care. In order to take account of these changes, the digital version of this chapter and the accompanying supplementary information available in the BSAVA Library will be updated as needed. Every effort has been made to ensure that the most up-to-date information has been included in this guide at the time of publication.

Pet obesity is a chronic medical condition with an increasing prevalence worldwide. A recent, large-scale study from veterinary clinics across North America, involving almost 5 million dogs and over 1 million cats (Montoya *et al.*, 2025), found that the prevalence of overweight and obese body condition increases with age, peaking at the mature adult life stage in both dogs (where 50.1% and 12.6% were in overweight and obese condition, respectively) and cats (where 44.8% and 21.7% were in overweight and obese condition, respectively). Although obese condition was uncommon, a significant proportion of growing kittens and puppies were in overweight condition during the late growth period (9.5% of puppies and 10.7% of kittens). This finding shows that cats and dogs, already in overweight or obese condition by this age, were significantly more likely to be so in adulthood (dogs: odds ratio 1.85; cats: odds ratio 1.52), suggesting that the impact on health can be lifelong.

Obesity is an insidious disease that develops as a result of a prolonged imbalance between energy consumed and energy used. There are many risk factors (Figure 15.1) and the pathogenesis is complex and interconnecting, making obesity a particularly challenging disease to manage. The prolonged state of positive energy balance leads to gradual expansion of white adipose tissue, both through hypertrophy (enlargement of existing adipocytes) and hyperplasia (increase in the number of adipocytes). Initially, the process can be considered as physiological (i.e. storing excess energy for future use) but continued expansion initiates pathological processes, such as adipose tissue hypoxia, provoking abnormal release of chemical mediators (so-called 'adipokines'). Adipose tissue can also be deposited around other organs, whilst adipocytes can infiltrate organ tissue itself, triggering dysregulation of metabolic, hormonal and inflammatory processes. This dysregulation is one of the mechanisms by which the adverse health consequences of obesity can arise.

Once obesity has developed, the only way it can be reversed is with caloric energy restriction, often coupled with increased physical activity (German *et al.*, 2007). Traditionally, this approach has required caloric restriction by feeding a dietetic diet designed for the purpose. Successful weight loss can take a prolonged period of time and may be challenging for the owner. Furthermore, even if the desired amount of weight is lost (a significant achievement), maintaining that loss can be a further challenge as maintenance energy requirements after weight loss are less than they were before

Category	Risk factor
Genetic	<ul><li>Deletion in the *pro-opiomelanocortin (POMC)* gene in Labrador and Flat-coated Retrievers is associated with appetite and weight gain (Raffan *et al.*, 2016)</li><li>Alternate allele of the *DENN* domain containing *1B (DENND1B)* gene is associated with obesity in Labrador Retrievers (Wallis *et al.*, 2025)</li><li>Obesity-prone breeds include Beagles, Cocker Spaniels, French Bulldogs, Golden Retrievers, Labrador Retrievers, Pugs and Rottweilers</li></ul>
Age	<ul><li>Rapid growth rate is associated with the future risk of obesity (Salt *et al.*, 2020)</li></ul>
Neutering	<ul><li>Neutering is associated with increased obesity risk</li></ul>
Other diseases	Positive associations with:<ul><li>Hyperadrenocorticism</li><li>Hypothyroidism</li><li>Insulinoma</li><li>Diseases affecting energy balance (e.g. orthopaedic disease affecting mobility)</li><li>Drug therapy (e.g. corticosteroids, anticonvulsants)</li></ul>
Environment and activity	Positive associations with:<ul><li>Indoor living</li><li>Low physical activity (frequency and duration)</li></ul>
Dietary factors	Positive associations with food type:<ul><li>Commercially manufactured dog foods</li><li>Dogs fed a mixture of commercially manufactured and homemade food are at greater risk of obesity than those fed one diet or the other</li></ul>Positive associations with feeding method:<ul><li>Offering food *ad libitum*</li><li>Once daily feeding</li><li>Feeding additional treats/snacks</li><li>Dogs present during food preparation</li><li>Using a scoop to measure food portions</li><li>Stealing food from other pets in the household</li><li>Owner sharing own food at mealtimes</li></ul>
Owner factors and behaviour	Positive associations with:<ul><li>Overweight status in dog and owner</li><li>Dogs living in an environment where the owner smokes</li><li>Close owner–dog bonds (e.g. tendency to 'over-humanize' dog, allowing dog to sleep on bed, seeing dog as 'a baby')</li><li>Owners using food as a reward</li></ul>Negative associations with:<ul><li>Interest in preventive healthcare for pet</li><li>Acceptance of obesity as a disease</li></ul>

Figure 15.1: Risk factors for canine obesity.

(German *et al.*, 2012a). Therefore, whilst obesity can often be managed, it can arguably never be cured, with some form of control likely being required for the rest of the life of the pet to prevent weight regain.

Different pathogenetic mechanisms link excess adiposity to health consequences; these are broadly grouped as 'mechanical' and 'chemical'. Mechanical effects are either the result of local deposition of adipose tissue that then impairs organ system function (e.g. respiratory compromise resulting from adipose tissue deposition in the thorax and neck affecting breathing) or increased overall body mass (e.g. additional bodyweight resulting in increased joint loading and affecting gait). Chemical mechanisms result from the production of adipokines and other molecules (i.e. cytokines, chemokines) within the adipose tissue, leading to inflammation, insulin resistance and impaired immune function (German *et al.*, 2010). There can be direct and indirect consequences of these pathogenetic mechanisms. Direct effects are those directly arising from impaired organ function, which can affect the ability of an animal to undertake normal daily activities; indirect effects are typically due to the development of other diseases (Figure 15.2) for which obesity is either a risk factor or exacerbator.

In dogs, obesity is associated with a shorter median lifespan, varying from 6 months to ≥2 years, depending on the breed (Salt *et al.*, 2018). In cats, the situation is more complicated as the optimal body condition score (BCS; see Figure 15.3) for lifespan and the optimal BCS for minimizing disease risk differ. Optimal lifespan effects are seen in cats with a BCS of 6/9. Animals with a BCS of <4/9 or 9/9 have been found to have a shorter lifespan than those cats with a BCS of 6/9 (Teng *et al.*, 2018a). Cats who reach a maximum BCS of 9/9 between 3 and 11 years of age also have on average a shorter lifespan. In contrast, to minimize the risk of disease development (e.g. musculoskeletal disease), the optimal BCS is 4–5/9, with an increased risk seen from a BCS of 6/9 upwards. Thus, in order to promote an optimal 'health span' (period of good quality of life), both lifespan (optimal BCS 6/9) and disease risk (optimal BCS 5/9) need to be taken into consideration (Teng *et al.*, 2018b). A BCS of 5–6/9 is currently recommended for cats. Both dogs and cats with obesity have a poorer quality of life, which can be alleviated with successful weight loss (German *et al.*, 2012b; Flanagan *et al.*, 2017; 2018).

Recent developments in the classification of obesity

In 2022, The Lancet tasked a commission of 58 international experts to provide a definition of obesity and to standardize diagnostic criteria in humans. The aim of the initiative was to enhance clinical decision-making and guide prioritization of therapeutic interventions. Following a review of the existing evidence and a consensus process, the commission published its findings in 2025 (Rubino *et al.*, 2025). The commission decided upon the following overarching definition of obesity, 'a condition characterized by excess adiposity, with or without abnormal distribution or function of adipose tissue, and with causes that are multifactorial and still incompletely understood'. The commission also proposed subdividing cases of obesity based on the presence of 'illness', defined as 'deviation from the healthy functioning of tissues, organs or the whole organism', into individuals with:

- **Clinical obesity** – 'a chronic, systemic illness characterized by alterations in the function of the tissues, organs, the entire individual, or a combination thereof, due to excess adiposity'
- **Preclinical obesity** – 'a state of excess adiposity with preserved function of other tissues and organs and a varying, but generally increased, risk of developing clinical obesity and several other non-communicable diseases'.

Disease category	Condition
Cardiorespiratory	■ Altered cardiovascular function ■ Brachycephalic airway obstruction syndrome ■ Decreased ventilation and oxygenation ■ Hypertension (mild) ■ Myocardial hypoxia ■ Tracheal collapse
Endocrine and metabolic	■ Diabetes mellitus, insulin resistance and obesity-related metabolic dysfunction ■ Hyperadrenocorticism ■ Hypothyroidism ■ Insulinoma
Gastrointestinal	■ Oral cavity disease ■ Pancreatitis
Musculoskeletal	■ Cruciate ligament disease ■ Hip dysplasia ■ Humeral condylar fractures ■ Intervertebral disc disease ■ Osteoarthritis
Neoplastic	■ Increased neoplasia risk ■ Mammary carcinoma ■ Transitional cell carcinoma
Urogenital	■ Abnormal urinary functional markers ■ Calcium oxalate urolithiasis ■ Glomerular disease ■ Lower urinary tract disease ■ Transitional cell carcinoma ■ Urethral sphincter mechanism incompetence
Other	■ Anaesthesia risk ■ Oxidative stress ■ Undesirable behaviours (aggression, nervousness, food-seeking and stealing, food guarding) ■ Poor skin and coat condition

Figure 15.2: Diseases for which obesity is either a risk factor or exacerbator in dogs.

As a result of this consensus in human medicine, changes to the way in which obesity is defined, classified and diagnosed in dogs and cats have been suggested (German *et al.*, 2025). Obesity in dogs and cats can be described as a condition characterized by excess adiposity, arising from multifactorial causes which, in some cases, can have both direct and indirect health consequences. Obesity can also be further classified as clinical or preclinical based on the degree to which the animal is affected:

■ **Clinical obesity** – a chronic illness resulting from alterations in organ or whole body function that are directly induced by excess adiposity, independent of the presence of other related diseases
■ **Preclinical obesity** – the presence of excess adiposity but without any clinical signs or functional impairments.

Diagnosing obesity

Classification of cases with obesity requires an assessment of both health and adiposity. In a primary care setting, adiposity is most commonly assessed using a combination of bodyweight measurement and BCS. A BCS assessment should be incorporated into a routine physical examination to provide a semi-quantitative evaluation of the degree of adiposity. Although many systems exist, the World Small Animal Veterinary Association (WSAVA) recommends use of the 9-point BCS system (Figure 15.3) (Freeman *et al.*, 2011). One limitation of this system is that some animals have marked obesity (>40% above ideal weight), which exceeds the maximum score (9/9). It can be difficult to determine the ideal weight in such patients and other methods are needed (e.g. historical weight recordings from the medical notes of the patient).

Whilst there is a positive correlation between bodyweight and body fat mass across a population, a single measurement is insufficient for an obesity diagnosis in an individual, not least in dogs where there is a diverse range of shapes and sizes across the breeds. However, bodyweight measurement has the advantage of being precise and accurate, particularly when the same set of scales (that are routinely calibrated) are used. Therefore, it can be useful as a longitudinal measure to assess changes in weight over time (e.g. for monitoring growth, for monitoring the outcomes of therapeutic weight reduction and for weight monitoring as part of an obesity prevention programme).

Veterinary professionals can assess the changes in bodyweight over time as evidence for a diagnosis of obesity when BCS is not available or an accurate assessment is not possible. For example, the current weight of the animal can be compared with a historical weight, ideally a measurement obtained during early adulthood. The basis for this method is that each BCS unit corresponds to approximately 10% additional weight (Laflamme, 1997; German *et al.*, 2006). Therefore, as long as the animal was not underweight at the time of the original measurement (this is unlikely if they were otherwise healthy and a young adult), a gain of 10–20% would suggest that the animal is in an overweight condition (BCS 6–7/9) or, possibly, in obese condition (BCS 8–9/9) if they were overweight at the time of the original assessment. Similarly, a weight gain of 20–40% would suggest that the animal is almost certainly in obese condition.

Individualized obesity care plan

Strategy

If possible, a team approach where cases are managed by a veterinary surgeon (veterinarian) and a veterinary nurse working together should be considered. If this is not possible, a veterinary nurse can oversee the majority of the care plan, but will require input from a veterinary surgeon about the classification of obesity (preclinical *versus* clinical), as well as the diagnosis and management of any obesity-related diseases.

Information gathering

Considerable information must be gathered and processed by the veterinary professional so that an individualized obesity care plan can be created for the pet. An in-depth approach should be adopted for the information gathering process, which may include the following:

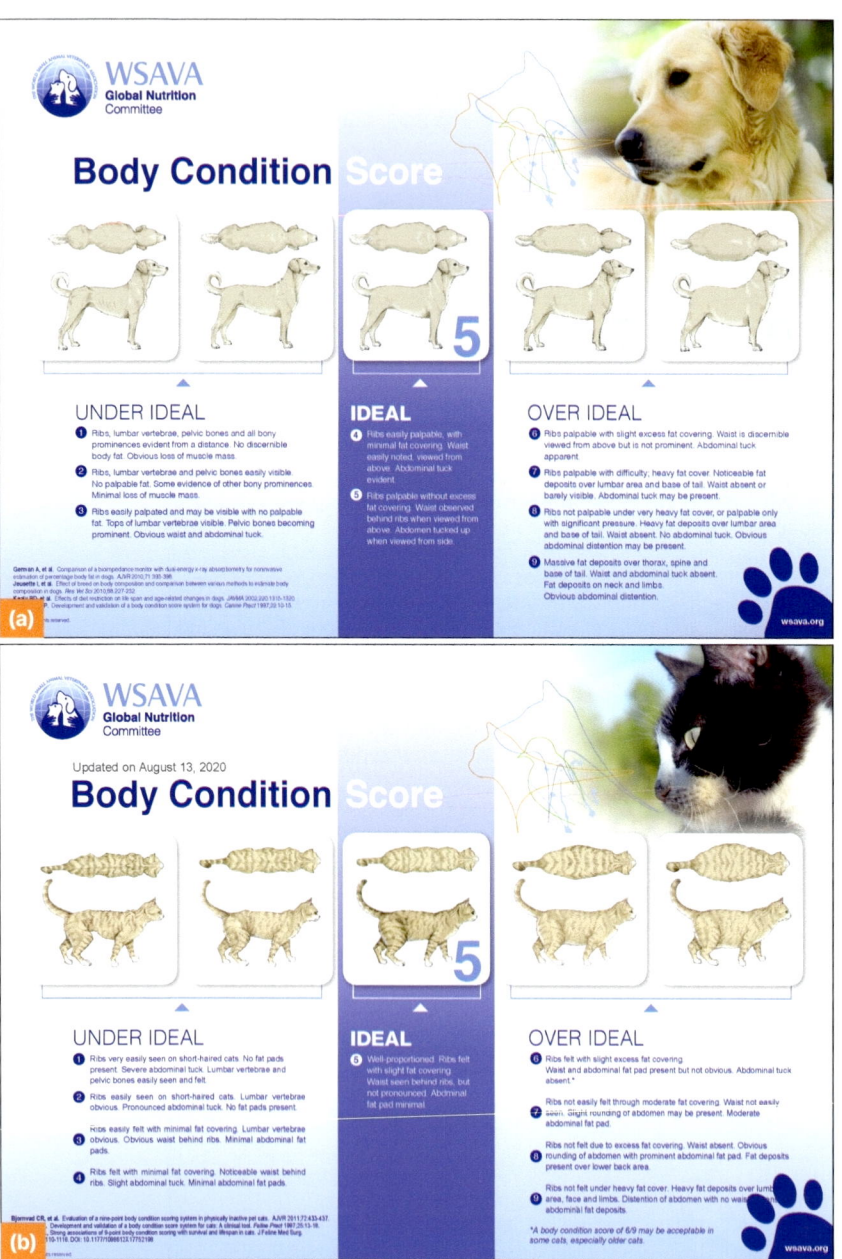

Figure 15.3: Body condition scoring chart for (a) dogs and (b) cats.
(Courtesy of the World Small Animal Veterinary Association).

- **Pre-appointment:**
  - Questionnaires on diet history and feeding management at home (paper or online)
  - A 3-day food diary
  - A review of previous clinical notes to ascertain:
    - Current and previous conditions or diseases
    - Dietary history
    - Evidence of gastrointestinal problems (to determine whether there may be problems with a dietary change)
    - Other relevant medical information (e.g. recent joint surgery that may affect ability to exercise, medication).
- **First appointment:**
  - Questions about feeding, food, lifestyle and family unit (e.g. how many members of the family are there?; is there a family member at home all day?; do you have a baby/young child?) typically covered by the veterinary nurse
  - Further questions (as needed) about the medical history to ascertain evidence of a direct impact of body fat on function, daily activities and quality of life. It a team approach is adopted, these questions could be asked by the veterinary surgeon.

A physical examination is then required and should include:

- Bodyweight measurement using calibrated scales appropriate for the size of the animal
- BCS assessment using a 9-point scale (see Figure 15.3)
- Muscle condition scoring using a 4-point system (see Chapter 11)
- Routine physical examination of all body systems (ideally undertaken by a veterinary surgeon in order to assess for the presence of other diseases and to identify possible functional effects directly associated with excess adipose tissue; e.g. altered patterns of breathing, panting, breathless when moving, alterations in movement and gait, poor skin and coat condition, pressure sores)
- Optional morphometric measurements (e.g. circumference of the neck, thorax (directly behind the forelimbs) and abdomen (at the waist)) obtained when the animal is standing
- Photography – photographs and videos of the pet from many different angles are beneficial for comparison as weight loss progresses (Figure 15.4). They are also a useful tool to celebrate successful weight loss when combined with pictures taken after the weight loss has been achieved.

Creating the care plan

Once all the information has been collected, it should be reviewed by the team and the goals and targets for the obesity care plan decided upon.

- **Goals** – broadly speaking, goals are something that the team are hoping to achieve (e.g. one or more intended improvements in health that should result from therapeutic weight reduction).
- **Targets** – these are specific weights (or other metrics) that can be set for different stages of the care plan (e.g. interim targets can be used to monitor progress and reinforce success in the eyes of the owner, and a final target weight at which point it is hoped that all the goals will have been achieved).

In addition to these goals and targets, an **ideal weight** (also known as a 'healthy weight') should be set. This is a weight point where the animal should be within the optimal body fat mass range, as determined by previous research and assessed by BCS.

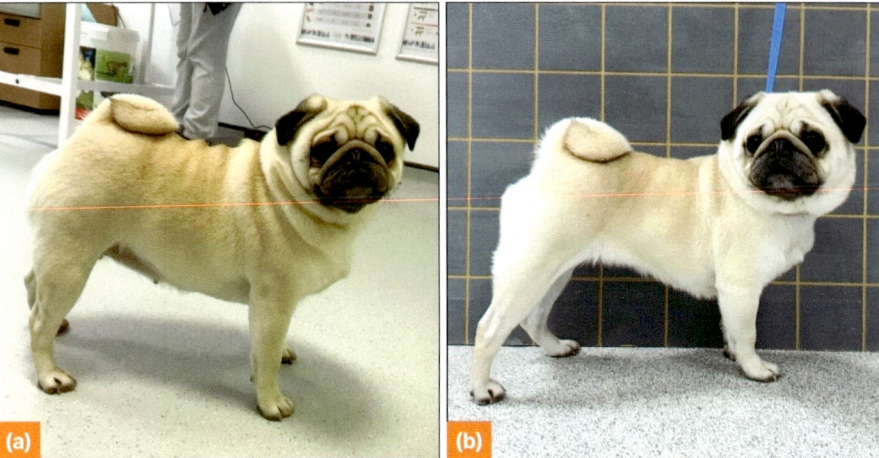

Figure 15.4: Photographs taken (a) before and (b) after weight loss can be useful to see the changes in body shape as weight loss progresses.
(© ROYAL CANIN® Obesity Care Clinic, University of Liverpool, UK).

The ideal weight needs to be determined because it is used as the basis for calculating daily food intake requirements. If either the current weight or target weight are used, this will lead to an erroneous (overestimated) daily food allocation, which may stifle progress and result in failure to lose weight, or even lead to weight gain.

When historical records are available, the best approach for determining the ideal weight is to identify an early adult bodyweight measurement (e.g. ideally when the animal was aged between 18 months and 2 years old) obtained when the animal was known to have been in optimal body condition (e.g. the recorded BCS was within the ideal range). If such information is not available, an ideal bodyweight can be approximated from the current weight and BCS by applying a correction factor (Figure 15.5); this correction factor assumes that each BCS unit equates to approximately 10% additional weight (Laflamme, 1997; German *et al.*, 2006).

Body condition score	Deviation above ideal weight	Calculation of ideal bodyweight
6	10%	Current bodyweight / 1.1
7	20%	Current bodyweight / 1.2
8	30%	Current bodyweight / 1.3
9	40%	Current bodyweight / 1.4

Figure 15.5: Calculation for determining ideal weight.

For some individuals, ideal weight and final target weight may be the same, especially young animals with no associated diseases. Thus, returning them to the optimal body fat range should maximize any benefits relating to lifespan and disease prevention. However, in some cases, the target weight set may not match the ideal weight (i.e. the target weight may be significantly greater). This type of plan would suit older animals (where lifestyle benefits associated with weight loss are less) and those individuals that already have associated diseases (as existing diseases cannot be prevented). The intention of therapeutic weight reduction in these animals is to improve function (in cases of clinical obesity), lessen the impact of any associated diseases and improve quality of life. Typically, only modest weight loss (6–9%) is necessary for such benefits to be seen (Marshall *et al.*, 2010; Flanagan *et al.*, 2017; 2018).

Once goals and targets have been established, and the ideal weight determined, this information can be used to create an individualized obesity care plan, which should include the following components:

- A summary of the formal diagnosis (clinical or preclinical obesity), degree of adiposity (BCS) and current bodyweight
- A summary of any obesity-associated diseases and other unrelated conditions (comorbidities)
- Details of goals, targets and ideal weight
- Diet choice for promoting therapeutic weight reduction
- Calculated daily food portion (based on ideal weight) and, if necessary, an estimate of daily cost
- Instructions about how to measure out food portions (i.e. using digital weighing scales and not measuring cups)
- Guidance about transitioning from the current diet to the food chosen for therapeutic weight reduction
- Instructions about how to feed the dog or cat, including the use of puzzle feeders, interactive food toys and automated feeders. The benefits of using a puzzle feeder include increasing activity, slowing consumption and providing mental stimulation
- Guidance about feeding any additional foods; although, it should be emphasized that deviation from the main meal dietary recommendation may hinder weight loss
    - The amount and type of additional food should be carefully selected. In this respect, vegetables can be recommended as a treat or when the pet is looking for additional food. These foods can also be used to add volume to each meal. Suitable vegetables include:
        - Courgette (for both cats and dogs)
        - Broccoli
        - Cauliflower
        - Cucumber
        - Green beans
        - Sprouts
        - Watermelon.
- A daily plan for physical activity outlining any adjustments required (e.g. walking, play behaviour and other activities). All recommendations should take into consideration the capabilities of both the owner and the pet, as well as other concurrent diseases (obesity-associated or unrelated)
- Other changes to lifestyle if recommended
- A summary of treatments needed to manage the consequences of clinical obesity or any other diseases that may be present
- A summary of the plan for monitoring and follow-up appointments
- Contact details should troubleshooting be required.

Monitoring the weight reduction phase of the care plan

During the initial stages of the obesity care plan, a review should be performed every 2–3 weeks to determine progress with the therapeutic weight reduction aspect of the plan. The primary measure for this is bodyweight (given the precision and accuracy) with zoometric measurements (tape measure readings), BCS assessment and photography only performed periodically (e.g. every 2–3 months). Changes in clinical condition should also be reviewed to determine progress with reference to the goals of the care plan.

If weight loss is progressing well, or the pet is distressed by travelling to the veterinary practice, the review interval can be extended to every 4 weeks, particularly during the later stages of the weight reduction phase. Cats and small dogs that are unable to attend the veterinary practice can be weighed at home using bathroom scales (the weight of the owner should be subtracted from the weight of the owner holding the animal), luggage scales (the weight of the carrier should be subtracted from the weight of the carrier with the animal placed inside) or baby/pet scales (if available). Although not as accurate as the weighing scales at the veterinary practice, this method still gives good guidance that weight loss is progressing. Ongoing support will be required throughout the process, and pet owners should have access to help via text, telephone or email between appointments.

The therapeutic weight reduction phase of an obesity can plan almost invariably takes longer than 3 months, and typically lasts many months or even years. Periodic rewards can help maintain owner motivation; for example, certificates can be awarded when interim targets are reached (Figure 15.6) with a more substantial reward given when the final target weight is achieved. It is preferable for such a reward to be positive for health (e.g. a toy to promote activity or a puzzle feeder). Other rewards such as rosettes or slimmer of the month can be given to acknowledge sustained hard work. Provided that the owner consents, before and after weight loss photographs can be displayed on the practice notice board, not only in celebration of achievement but also to inspire other pet owners to enrol.

Reaching target weight and monitoring during the maintenance phase

Like in humans, weight regain is frequently observed in pets, with approximately half of dogs and cats that successfully reach their target weight regaining some or all of the weight that has been lost (German *et al.*, 2012a; Deagle *et al.*, 2014). To avoid this, the obesity care plan should also include guidance for the maintenance phase. Many of the strategies used during therapeutic weight reduction can be adapted for this phase, including measuring food portions accurately, minimizing the amount of additional food provided and promoting physical activity. The main difference is that food intake needs to be adjusted to ensure that bodyweight stabilizes and is maintained long term. The following approach can be used to transition between the weight reduction and maintenance phases:

1. Increase food intake by a small amount (e.g. approximately 5%) and reweigh the animal after 2 weeks.
2. If there is continuing weight loss at the first follow-up visit, increase food intake by approximately 5% and reweigh after a further 2 weeks.
3. If weight has been regained at the first follow-up visit, decrease food intake by half the amount it was originally increased by (e.g. approximately 2.5%) and reweigh after a further 2 weeks.
4. Repeat the process of adjustments (i.e. further small increases or decreases) and fortnightly checks until weight is stable.

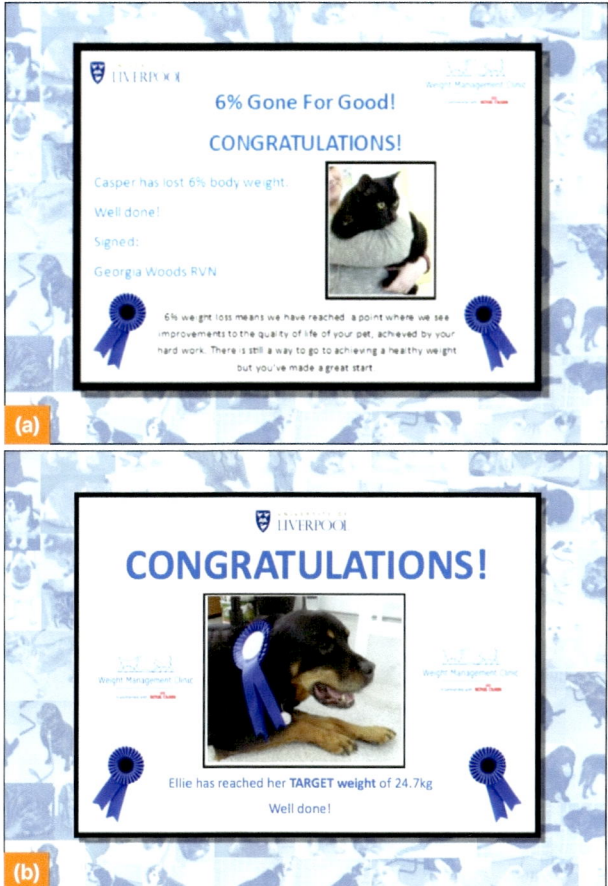

Figure 15.6: Certificates can be used to (a) reward stages of weight loss and (b) celebrate achieving target weight loss.
(© ROYAL CANIN® Obesity Care Clinic, University of Liverpool, UK).

5. Continue with regular weight checks long term. Gradually increase the interval between the checks (e.g. every 4 weeks, every 8 weeks and then every 3 months) provided that weight continues to remain stable.
6. Thereafter, continue to weigh the animal regularly (at least every 6 months, but more often if possible).

Unless a different medical condition necessitates it, the dietetic food used for the weight reduction phase should continue to be fed for the maintenance phase. Compared with switching to a different food (e.g. a standard or even 'light' maintenance diet), the risk of weight regain is significantly less when the diet used for the reduction phase is continued (German *et al.*, 2012a).

The effect of nutrition

An appropriate diet is critical to ensure that the process of therapeutic weight reduction is safe. The key components of a dietetic food for weight loss include:

- **Being complete and balanced:**
  - The diet must deliver all essential nutrients to the pet in the correct quantities, during both the weight reduction and maintenance phases. In dietetic food that has been formulated to facilitate therapeutic weight reduction, concentrations of essential nutrients are increased, relative to the energy content of the diet, ensuring that all needs are met even in the face of caloric restriction. It is inadvisable to use a diet that has not been formulated for such a purpose, as the degree of energy restriction required puts the dog or cat at risk of developing nutrient deficiencies (Linder *et al.*, 2012).
- **Energy restriction:**
  - Energy restriction is required to facilitate therapeutic weight reduction by creating a negative energy balance. Different strategies should be considered depending on the degree of obesity:
    - Should the pet have a BCS of 6/9 in dogs or 7/9 in cats (i.e. <10% above its ideal weight), a short-term (8–12 weeks) period of weight reduction can be attempted using a low-energy (e.g. light) maintenance diet (Keller *et al.*, 2020). However, there is a limit to the degree of energy restriction that can safely be used with such a diet; 80% of maintenance requirements (based on ideal weight) being the lower limit. If no weight loss is observed when using a low-energy maintenance diet fed at this level, a purpose-formulated dietetic weight reduction food is instead needed
    - Should the pet have a BCS of >6/9 in dogs or >7/9 in cats (i.e. ≥20% above its ideal weight), dietetic food formulated for weight loss is always recommended, given that a greater degree of energy restriction is needed for a much longer period of time.
- **Minimizing food-seeking behaviours:**
  - A major challenge and reason for weight loss failure, is that restricting food intake leads to hunger which causes food-seeking behaviours (e.g. stealing food or bothering the owner for food). Dietetic foods can be modified to promote satiety, mitigating some these problem behaviours. One approach is to modify the macronutrient content (e.g. increase the protein and fibre content) (Weber *et al.*, 2007; Bissot *et al.*, 2010) and, if using a dry food, to alter the shape of the kibble (Sagols *et al.*, 2019). The basis for these modifications are:
    - **Increased fibre content** – an increased concentration of fibre in the diet increases gastric volume and delays gastric emptying. Both improve feelings of fullness and help to reduce food-seeking behaviours. This modification is most effective in dogs; whilst there is some effect in cats, over-supplementation with fibre can adversely affect palatability
    - **Increased protein content** – in dogs, increased dietary protein improves satiety, decreasing voluntary food intake with no loss of palatability. However, in cats, increased dietary protein actually increases food intake (Bissot *et al.*, 2010); therefore, whilst protein supplementation is necessary to minimize lean tissue loss, the exact amount of supplementation needs to be carefully titrated
    - **Kibble shape** – changing the shape of a kibble can affect the amount of chewing that is required and improve satiety; the effect is a modest decrease in voluntary food intake.

■ **Provision of feeding method options:**
- The diet should be able to be used with slow feeder bowls (Figure 15.7) or interactive feeding toys (Figure 15.8), as these increase meal duration and might contribute to improvements in satiety.

■ **Management of treats:**
- Ideally, owners should be instructed to stop providing any high calorie foods as treats. These may include:
  - Pre-packaged or homemade treats
  - Rewards (e.g. training treats)
  - Human foods and drinks (e.g. milk, scraps, leftovers)
  - Dental chews or anything given for teeth cleaning. Brushing with an appropriate toothbrush and pet-friendly toothpaste should be encouraged instead
  - Rawhide chews
  - Cooked or uncooked animal bones.
- Given how important it is that owners reward their pet with a food treat, most owners will not accept the advice that treats need to be stopped altogether. Instead, alternative options should be proposed; examples of suitable options include:
  - Reserving part of the daily allowance of dry food
  - Courgette (also known as zucchini) can be given to both cats and dogs; for cats the skin should be removed and it should be cooked by steaming or microwaving
  - Broccoli
  - Cauliflower
  - Green beans
  - Sprouts
  - Watermelon
  - Cucumber.

■ **Wet and dry food options:**
- To allow a pet's preferences and routines to be met.

■ **Palatable:**
- Pets must want to consume the food offered. Palatability is vital for overall success.

■ **Easy to obtain:**
- Not all pet owners can travel to the veterinary practice every few weeks to obtain food, especially if large bags are desired or the owner does not have their own means of transport. Nor can all pet owners order food online. The dietary recommendation must be easily obtainable for the owner in the long term.

> **Note:** The term 'begging' has negative associations and refers to the actions of humans; 'food-seeking behaviour' is the preferred term for behaviours displayed by dogs and cats.

Essential elements

In addition to dietary alterations, other aspects are required to maximize the chances of success of the obesity care plan.

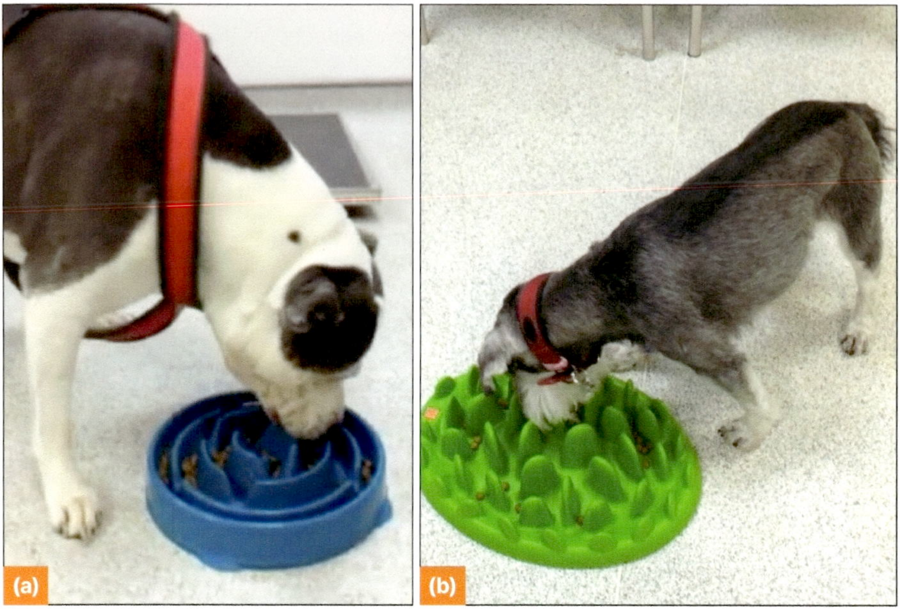

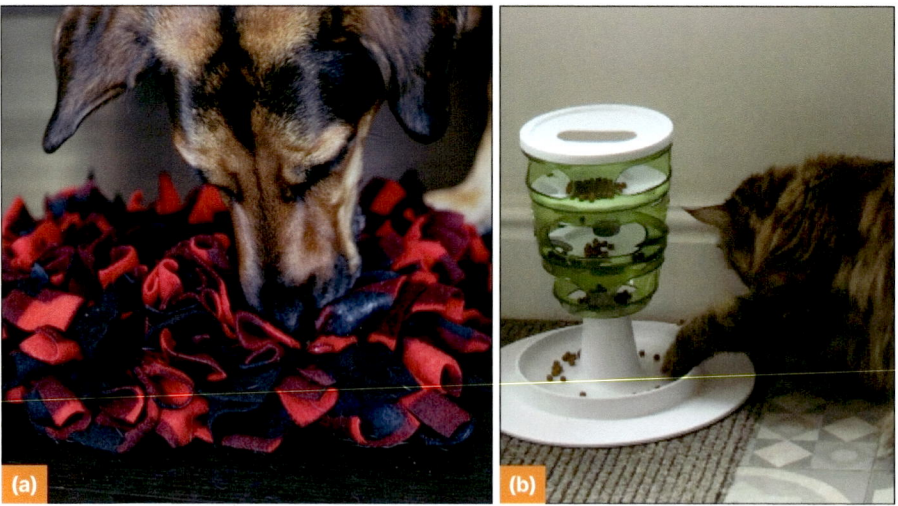

Figure 15.7: There are various types of slow feeder pet bowls available including (a) a maze type and (b) a grass type with varying sizes of vertical sections.
(© ROYAL CANIN® Obesity Care Clinic, University of Liverpool, UK).

Figure 15.8: Interactive feeding toys can be useful for feeding pets. (a) Snuffle mat and (b) food tower.
(a, Image used under the licence from Shutterstock.com: © Tonia Kraakman; b, © Georgia Woods-Lee).

Routine monitoring and recording of weight and body condition score for all patients

Weighing and performing a BCS assessment (every pet at every point of contact) and recording the results in patient's record is useful for obesity prevention strategies, as well as for building up a historical record should it be required in the future (e.g. to determine an ideal weight should obesity care subsequently be needed). In this way, changes to bodyweight and BCS can be identified early, enabling corrective measures to be implemented.

System of referral for patients with obesity

Many patients with obesity will be diagnosed through regular weighing and BCS assessment. The practice will need to have a system in place to deal efficiently with such cases. Ideally, a team approach should be considered, with one or two staff members taking primary responsibility (e.g. a veterinary nurse and a veterinary surgeon) for providing obesity care, assessing cases, setting goals and targets, and then implementing and monitoring plans. Thus, when a patient with obesity is identified, the practice should have a system for internally referring them to those team members for care.

Diet choices for obesity care

Suitable diets

Suitable diet choices include:

- Commercially produced dietetic food specifically formulated for feeding at a reduced level of energy intake (e.g. during both the therapeutic weight reduction phase and the subsequent maintenance phase). These diets will have been designed to ensure that essential nutrient requirements are still met despite the reduced intake (German et al., 2015)
- Home-prepared cooked diets (see Chapter 5) might also be suitable, but only if the recipe is designed and overseen by an appropriately qualified individual (see Chapter 1). Typically, these diets include appropriate vitamin and mineral supplementation.

Unsuitable diets

Unsuitable diet choices include:

- Any diet that has not been formulated to be complete and balanced when fed for a prolonged period of time for therapeutic weight reduction and beyond (e.g. a diet formulated to meet maintenance requirements only)
- Any diet containing uncooked ingredients (see Chapter 6) that has not been formulated and overseen by an appropriately qualified individual. Such diets are uniquely difficult to balance and increase the risk of nutrient deficiencies even when fed at maintenance levels. Deliberately feeding such a diet at a level considerably below maintenance requirements dramatically increases the risk and cannot be recommended.

Diets that align with pet preferences and owner routine

Never change more than is necessary to make progress in a particular case. For this reason, it is best to choose a diet type (wet, dry or a combination) that suits the preferences of the pet.

Other management factors

Obesity care for senior pets or those with concurrent disease

Obesity care plans should still be considered for older pets and those with comorbidities. The targets set in these cases should be tailored to the likely benefits to health. Measurable improvements in mobility and quality of life can be seen after only a small amount of weight loss, therefore, the aim should be to induce the minimum amount of weight loss necessary to achieve the goals (Marshall *et al.*, 2010; Flanagan *et al.*, 2017; 2018). The majority (approximately 83%) of body tissue that is lost during the weight reduction process is fat, although some lean tissue is also lost, with the amount increasing as the percentage of weight loss increases (German, 2016). Excessive lean tissue loss is undesirable, especially in senior patients and those with comorbidities since outcomes can be adversely affected. Patients should be monitored closely throughout the process.

Senior age

For dogs and cats with obesity who are in the senior life stage, a weight reduction of 10–15% should be sufficient for quality of life and mobility improvements, without negative consequences (see Chapter 11).

Chronic kidney disease

The severity of chronic kidney disease (CKD) can be categorized using the International Renal Interest Society (IRIS) staging system. Therapeutic weight reduction can be safely undertaken in cats and dogs who are at IRIS stage 1 or 2 CKD (provided that the serum phosphate concentration is <1.5 mmol/l); as with senior cats and dogs, a maximum of 10–15% loss is generally recommended, since greater amounts of weight loss can cause excessive lean tissue loss. Although dietetic foods for weight reduction typically have an increased protein and, therefore, phosphorus content, they can still be used (for the weight reduction phase only) because any increase in daily phosphorus intake (from the increased amount in the food) is offset by the decreased daily food intake (since the animal is fed approximately 60% of the maintenance energy requirement; see Chapter 2). However, when transitioning from the weight reduction to the maintenance phase, a different diet should be used; for example, a senior diet (with a modest amount of phosphorus restriction) or a low phosphorus dietetic food designed for animals with CKD (see Chapter 19).

Orthopaedic disease

In these cases, improved mobility is always desirable. Measurable improvements may be demonstrated after just 6–9% weight loss (Marshall *et al.*, 2010). As these animals have limitations in terms of the physical activity they can undertake, it is sensible to restrict their daily intake by approximately 5% more than the typical starting amount (for their ideal weight, sex and neutering status).

Misconceptions about pet obesity

Pet obesity is all the owner's fault

Obesity is a complex disease and, although owners have some control over what their pet eats and how much they exercise, there are many other factors outside of their control (e.g. genetic and environmental influences). Given the multitude of (often overlapping) factors, it is both wrong and unhelpful to blame the owner for the development of obesity in their pet.

Pets with obesity can be healthy

Although pets with obesity may appear to be fit and healthy, particularly from the point of view of the owner, direct effects of obesity can often be identified on close questioning, and they are still at risk of developing associated diseases. Since these health consequences take time to develop, the absence of concurrent problems can be used as an incentive to actively maintain health.

Obesity can be managed through exercise alone

Increasing physical activity alone is ineffective as a therapeutic weight reduction strategy (Chapman *et al.*, 2019) and owners who attempt to achieve weight loss in their pet simply by increasing exercise are rarely successful. Therefore, dietary management should always be used, and this can be successful even in patients with limited mobility. Nonetheless, whenever feasible, adding physical activity to the plan is recommended because this can help to preserve lean tissue (Vitger *et al.*, 2016).

Preventing obesity

Arguably, preventing obesity is more important than waiting for it to develop and then implementing a therapeutic weight reduction plan. Despite this, prevention strategies are rarely considered by veterinary professionals. Adipose tissue accumulates progressively, starting early in life (including during the growth phase in some individuals) and, once developed, can be immensely difficult to correct. Therefore, preventing obesity can be a challenge and an organized strategy involving the entire veterinary team is required. Any strategy needs to be proactive, cover the entire lifespan of the dog or cat and be implemented early in life, ideally at the first vaccination consultation.

The key stage of an obesity prevention strategy is the early-life period (i.e. puppyhood or kittenhood; see Chapter 10). Implementation of the prevention strategy during this life stage ensures that any interventions can commence early, hopefully before the problem has started. In order to achieve this, the potential of an individual dog or cat developing obesity should be determined based on known risk factors (see Figure 15.1). It is recommended that regular weight measurements should be obtained throughout the development period and used to monitor the pattern of growth against validated growth standards (see Chapter 10). If the growth pattern of a particular animal is seen to deviate from optimal (e.g. crossing centile lines upwards or downwards), possible reasons should be investigated and changes implemented (e.g. decreasing the amount of food provided). The success of these changes can then be determined at follow-up weight checks.

Once the dog or cat reaches skeletal maturity (see Chapter 10), their body condition should be verified and, if determined to be in ideal condition, the concurrent weight can be recorded as their 'healthy adult weight' (the weight they should aim to maintain throughout their adult life). This 'healthy adult weight' can, therefore, act as a reference weight for any future visits, with the main goal being to maintain bodyweight within ±5% of this reference weight. This weight can also be used as the 'ideal' bodyweight should obesity develop and a therapeutic weight reduction plan be needed. From this point onwards, regular weight measurements should be obtained at least annually, or more frequently if possible. Compliance with such a monitoring strategy can be improved if weight checks coincide with other preventive medicine visits (e.g. for vaccination, deworming, microchipping) or routine health checks.

Communication with pet owners

Many veterinary professionals struggle communicating with owners about obesity due to concerns about causing offence. However, it is rare for owners to react in this way, and it is critical that these conversations take place in order for the dog or cat to benefit from appropriate obesity care and the health improvements that therapeutic weight reduction will bring. Strategies to facilitate obesity conversations include:

- Measuring bodyweight and assessing BCS for **every** patient at **every** visit, and ensuring that the findings are recorded in the patient's record:
  - By routinely performing these measurements, owners will understand what they mean and the importance of their pet maintaining a healthy weight. Introducing such assessments when the pet is an ideal weight makes it easier to subsequently discuss weight
  - Bodyweight and BCS can be used as proxies for obesity when holding discussions with owners (not least during the initial consultation when it is not known how an owner will react). The veterinary professional can discuss changes in weight and BCS (e.g. increases above the healthy weight of the animal) without terms such as 'obesity' or 'overweight' having to be used.
- Using BCS assessment as a method of initiating a conversation about weight:
  - Owners can easily be shown how to conduct a BCS assessment on their pet and, in doing so (with a little guidance and encouragement), may realize that their pet is overweight. By recognizing this for themselves they may be more likely to accept the information.
- Discussing the risks of excess adiposity, relating them wherever possible to any other clinical concerns:
  - Owners may struggle to associate the signs they observe in their pet (e.g. mobility issues, snoring and other respiratory signs) with obesity; convincing owners of such a link might improve the likelihood that they will accept a weight reduction plan. Making owners aware of other possible disease risks can sometimes also be persuasive.
- Talking to the pet, not the owner!
  - If the communication style adopted during the consultation involves 'chatting' to the pet as they are being examined, the topic of weight gain can be introduced whilst the cat or dog is on the scales. This can help to gauge the readiness of the owner to have a conversation about obesity and allow the veterinary professional to act accordingly.

All conversations about obesity should be constructive and supportive, whilst avoiding blame which can be counterproductive. Care should also be taken not to devalue the importance or impact of this disease with the use of humorous or derogatory terms with negative connotations, which might cause offence. Rarely is attempting to shock the owner into action well received. Finally, although the terms 'overweight' and 'obese' are the formal terminology, owners may have negative associations with these words; therefore, phrases such as 'above ideal weight' or 'above a healthy weight' are preferable (especially if the practice adopts the approach of setting a 'healthy adult weight').

Conclusion

Pet obesity is a complex and challenging disease to manage, and lifelong care is often required for affected individuals. Tailored obesity care plans with the main priority of improving quality of life should be used, and the veterinary team should work with the owner to motivate them as much as possible along the weight loss journey of their pet.

References and further reading

Bissot T, Servet E, Vidal S *et al.* (2010) Novel dietary strategies can improve the outcome of weight loss programmes in obese client-owned cats. *Journal of Feline Medicine and Surgery* **12**, 104–112

Chapman M, Woods GRT, Ladha C, Westgarth C and German AJ (2019) An open-label randomised clinical trial to compare the efficacy of dietary caloric restriction and physical activity for weight loss in overweight pet dogs. *Veterinary Journal* **243**, 65–73

Courcier EA, O'Higgins R, Mellor DJ and Yam PS (2010) Prevalence and risk factors for feline obesity in a first opinion practice in Glasgow, Scotland. *Journal of Feline Medicine and Surgery* **12**, 746–753

Daley A, Jolly K, Madigan C *et al.* (2019) A brief behavioural intervention to promote regular self-weighing to prevent weight regain after weight loss: a RCT. *Public Health Research* **7**, 1–66

Deagle G, Holden SL, Biourge V, Morris PJ and German AJ (2014) Long-term follow-up after weight management in obese cats. *Journal of Nutritional Science* **3**, DOI: 10.1017/jns.2014.36

Deagle G, Holden SL, Biourge V, Queau Y and German AJ (2015) The kinetics of weight loss in obese client-owned cats. In: *BSAVA Congress Proceedings 2015* p. 491

Deagle G, Holden SL, Biourge V, Serisier S and German AJ (2015) The kinetics of weight loss in obese client-owned dogs: ESVCN-O-1. *Journal of Veterinary Internal Medicine* **29**, 443–444

Donataccio MP, Vanzo A and Bosello O (2021) Obesity paradox and heart failure. *Eating and Weight Disorders* **26**, 1697–1707

Flanagan J, Bissot T, Hours MA, Moreno B, Feugier A and German AJ (2017) Success of a weight loss plan for overweight dogs: the results of an international weight loss study. *PLoS One* **12(9)**, DOI: 10.1371/ journal.pone.0184199

Flanagan J, Bissot T, Hours MA, Moreno B and German AJ (2018) An international multi-centre cohort study of weight loss in overweight cats: differences in outcome in different geographical locations. *PLoS One* **13(7)**, DOI: 10.1371/journal. pone.0200414

Foster GD, Wadden TA, Makris AP *et al.* (2003) Primary care physicians' attitudes about obesity and its treatment. *Obesity Research* **11**, 1168–1177

Freeman L, Becvarova I, Cave N *et al.* (2011) WSAVA Nutritional Assessment Guidelines. *Journal of Small Animal Practice* **52**, 385–396

German AJ (2006) The growing problem of obesity in dogs and cats. *Journal of Nutrition* **136(7)**, 1940S–1946S

German AJ (2016) Weight management in obese pets: the tailoring concept and how it can improve results. *Acta Veterinaria Scandinavica* **58**, 3–9

German AJ, Holden SL, Bissot T, Hackett RM and Biourge V (2007) Dietary energy restriction and successful weight loss in obese client-owned dogs. *Journal of Veterinary Internal Medicine* **21**, 1174–1180

German AJ, Holden SL, Mason SL *et al.* (2011) Imprecision when using measuring cups to weigh out extruded dry kibbled food. *Journal of Animal Physiology and Animal Nutrition* **95**, 368–373

German AJ, Holden SL, Morris PJ and Biourge V (2012a) Long-term follow-up after weight management in obese dogs: the role of diet in preventing regain. *Veterinary Journal* **192**, 65–70

German AJ, Holden SL, Moxham GL, *et al.* (2006) A simple, reliable tool for owners to assess the body condition of their dog or cat. *The Journal of Nutrition* **136(7 Suppl)**, 2031S–2033S

German AJ, Holden SL, Serisier S *et al.* (2015) Assessing the adequacy of essential nutrient intake in obese dogs undergoing energy restriction for weight loss: a cohort study. *BMC Veterinary Research* **11**, 253

German AJ, Holden SL, Wiseman-Orr ML *et al.* (2012b) Quality of life is reduced in obese dogs but improves after successful weight loss. *Veterinary Journal* **192**, 428–434

German AJ, Ryan VH, German AC, Wood IS and Trayhurn P (2010) Obesity, its associated disorders and the role of inflammatory adipokines in companion animals. *Veterinary Journal* **185**, 4–9

German AJ, Woods GRT, Holden SL, Brennan L and Burke C (2018) Dangerous trends in pet obesity. *Veterinary Record* **182**, 25–25

German AJ, Woods GRT, Ward E and Churchill J (2025) We should adopt new definitions for clinical obesity in companion animals. *Veterinary Record* **196**, 197–198

Gravina G, Ferrari F and Nebbiai G (2021) The obesity paradox and diabetes. *Eating and Weight Disorders* **26**, 1057–1068

Keller E, Sagols E, Flanagan J, Biourge V and German AJ (2020) Use of reduced-energy content maintenance diets for modest weight reduction in overweight cats and dogs. *Research in Veterinary Science* **131**, 194–205

Kopelman PG (2000) Obesity as a medical problem. *Nature* **404**, 635–643

Laflamme D (1997) Development and validation of a body condition score system for dogs. *Canine Practice* **22**, 10–15

Linder DE, Freeman LM, Morris P *et al.* (2012) Theoretical evaluation of risk for nutritional deficiency with calorie restriction in dogs. *Veterinary Quarterly* **32**, 123–129

Marshall WG, Hazewinkel HAW, Mullen D *et al.* (2010) The effect of weight loss on lameness in obese dogs with osteoarthritis. *Veterinary Research Communications* **34**, 241–253

Martinez-Tapia C, Diot T, Oubaya N *et al.* (2021) The obesity paradox for mid- and long-term mortality in older cancer patients: a prospective multicenter cohort study. *American Journal of Clinical Nutrition* **113**, 129–141

Montoya M, Péron F, Hookey T *et al.* (2025) Overweight and obese body condition in ~4.9 million dogs and ~1.3 million cats seen at primary practices across the USA: prevalences by life stage from early growth to senior. *Preventative Veterinary Medicine* **235**, 106398

Pearl RL, Wadden TA, Bach C, Leonard SM and Michel KE (2020) Who's a good boy? Effects of dog and owner body weight on veterinarian perceptions and treatment recommendations. *International Journal of Obesity* **44**, 2455–2464

Raffan E, Dennis RJ, O'Donovan CJ *et al.* (2016) A deletion in the canine POMC gene is associated with weight and appetite in obesity-prone Labrador Retriever dogs. *Cell Metabolism* **23(5)**, 893–900

Rubino F, Cummings DE, Eckel RH *et al.* (2025) Definition and diagnostic criteria of clinical obesity. *The Lancet Diabetes and Endocrinology* **13(3)**, 221–262

Sagols E, Hours MA, Daniel I *et al.* (2019) Comparison of the effects of different kibble shape on voluntary food intake and palatability of weight loss diets in pet dogs. *Research in Veterinary Science* **124**, 375–382

Salt C, Morris PJ, Butterwick RF *et al.* (2020) Comparison of growth patterns in healthy dogs and dogs in abnormal body condition using growth standards. *PLoS One* **15(9)**, e0238521

Salt C, Morris PJ, Wilson D, Lund EM and German AJ (2018) Association between lifespan and canine body condition: an epidemiological study in neutered client-owned dogs. *Journal of Veterinary Internal Medicine* **33**, 89–99

Slupe JL, Freeman LM and Rush JE (2008) Association of body weight and body condition with survival in dogs with heart failure. *Journal of Veterinary Internal Medicine* **22**, 561–565

Teng KT, McGreevy PD, Toribio JL *et al.* (2018a) Strong associations of nine-point body condition scoring with survival and lifespan in cats. *Journal of Feline Medicine and Surgery* **20(12)**, 1110–1118

Teng KT, McGreevy PD, Toribio JL *et al.* (2018b) Associations of body condition score with health conditions related to overweight and obesity in cats. *Journal of Small Animal Practice* **59**, 603–615

Thorne CJ (1982) Feeding behaviour in the cat – recent advances. *Journal of Small Animal Practice* **23**, 555–562

Vitger AD, Stallknecht BM, Nielsen DH and Bjornvad CR (2016) Integration of a physical training program in a weight loss plan for overweight pet dogs. *Journal of the American Veterinary Medical Association* **248**, 174–182

Wallis NJ, McClellan A, Mörseburg A *et al.* (2025) Canine genome-wide association study identifies *DENND1B* as an obesity gene in dogs and humans. *Science* **387**, DOI: 10.1126/science.ads2145

Weber M, Bissot T, Servet E *et al.* (2007) A high-protein, high-fiber diet designed for weight loss improves satiety in dogs. *Journal of Veterinary Internal Medicine* **21**, 1203–1208

Online extras

This chapter includes:

- **A client information leaflet that is available to download and print from the BSAVA Library**

Access via QR code or: bsavalibrary.com/nutrition_15

Restricted activity

16

Restricted activity may be pet-led (e.g. due to ageing), prescribed by a veterinary professional to allow for recovery from injury or surgery (Figure 16.1), or required for the management of a long-term disease (Figure 16.2). Restricted activity can be instigated for a short period of time (e.g. just a few days or weeks following a surgical procedure) or be much longer in duration (e.g. months or years for ongoing orthopaedic concerns). No matter what the duration or motivation for restriction, nutritional adjustments should be considered.

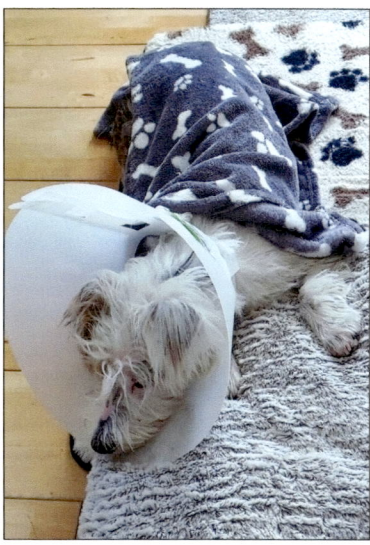

Figure 16.1: Dog with restricted activity to allow recovery from surgery.
(Courtesy of Sam Britton)

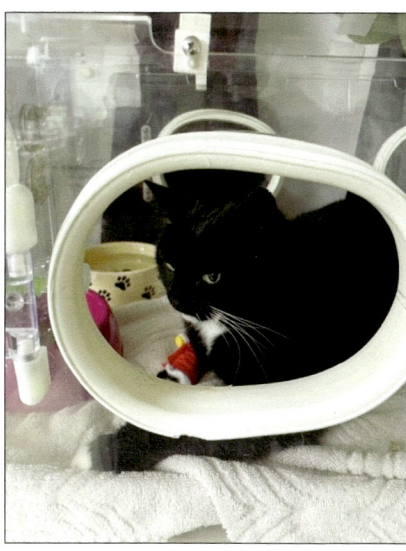

Figure 16.2: Cat with restricted activity during a stay in hospital for management of a long-term disease.
(Courtesy of Sam Britton)

The maintenance energy requirement (MER) (see Chapter 2) is the amount of energy a pet requires each day to perform all their usual daily activities whilst keeping their weight stable. In the presence of disease or injury, additional energy is occasionally required for healing and recovery. However, during these times activity is often restricted meaning that the energy expended on daily activities is decreased. These factors do not cancel each other out as the additional energy required for healing and recovery is, in most cases, minor or non-existent. Thus, the reduction in normal activity can often affect the MER profoundly. If no dietary alterations are made, there may be an unwanted gain in adipose tissue as the result of a positive energy state, predisposing the pet to obesity (see Chapter 15). Obesity adversely affects quality of life and, together with other concurrent diseases, can cause many negative effects. Therefore, it is critical to adjust food intake to prevent such negative consequences.

The effect of nutrition

Nutrition plays a key role in promoting health and preventing weight gain during times of restricted activity. Optimal nutrition should be provided throughout the period of restricted activity, with delivery of all nutrients in the appropriate quantities. The nutritional recommendation will depend on species, age, level of restriction, expected duration of restriction and concurrent medical problems. The patient should be monitored carefully throughout the period of restricted activity. Completing a nutritional assessment as early as possible during the period of activity restriction will highlight points of concern. Owners should also be asked to complete a food diary for their pet during this time. These measures, together with regular weight checks, should allow good control of nutritional intake and prevention of weight gain.

Essential elements

Dietary alterations and considerations when instigating activity restriction include:

- **Short-term activity restriction:** 7–10 days (e.g. postoperative period following neutering)
  - Care should be taken to reduce feeding extra food (e.g. treats and snacks) or replace them with calorie appropriate alternatives during this time
  - Good quality complete and balanced diets should be fed
  - Cats and dogs should be weighed following the period of restricted activity to ensure unintended weight gain has not occurred; if it has occurred, alterations to the diet may be needed
  - All food allocations should be calculated for the pet owner to ensure the correct amounts are being fed
  - All food allocations should be weighed out carefully on digital scales each day to prevent over- or underfeeding.
- **Mid-term activity restriction:** 4–6 weeks (e.g. following fracture repair)
  - Cats and dogs should be weighed regularly throughout this time (e.g. every 2 weeks) and action quickly taken to restabilize the weight if changes are observed
  - Care should be taken to eliminate all treats, snacks and food extras (or to replace them with calorie appropriate alternatives) during this time
  - Part of the daily food allowance could be used as rewards
  - Good quality complete and balanced diets should be fed
  - All food (and treat) allocations should be calculated for the pet owner to ensure the correct amounts are being fed
  - All food allocations should be weighed on digital scales each day to prevent over- or underfeeding
  - A reduced calorie diet may be used (e.g. a 'light' diet could be recommended to provide a small overall calorie reduction). It is important to note that 'light' diets are not suitable for therapeutic weight reduction in most cases. For a pet up to 10%

above their optimal weight, a 'light' diet may be used in the short term, but for no longer than 8 weeks, as the risk of nutritional deficiencies increase after this time if nutrient concentrations are too restricted (Keller *et al.*, 2020)
- Obesity care should be initiated if required. Recovery will not be compromised provided suitable weight loss diets are used. All specifically formulated weight loss diets should deliver complete and balanced nutrition with only the calorie content restricted (see Chapter 15)
- Therapeutic diets for controlled weight reduction could be fed during this time, regardless of whether obesity is present or not (e.g. if the dog or cat is prone to obesity). In such cases, food-seeking behaviours can be challenging, but there are several components of therapeutic diets that can help alleviate such behaviour (e.g. expanded kibbles, increased fibre content)
- Alleviation of boredom. Often very active pets struggle when their activity is restricted and can display negative behaviours (see below).
- **Long-term activity restriction:** over 6 weeks (e.g. cases of osteoarthritis)
  - Pets in this category are at high risk of developing obesity if alterations to the diet are not made
  - All points listed above for mid-term activity restriction should be followed but for a longer duration of time
  - Activity within the limits of the pet should be encouraged. This may include the use of puzzle toys or slow feeder food bowls, which increase general activity without risking injury.

Hydrotherapy (a form of non-weight bearing activity) can be instigated if appropriate (Figure 16.3). Reputable providers of hydrotherapy should be sought. Ideally, patients should be referred to a centre where the hydrotherapist is a member of the Association of Chartered Physiotherapists in Animal Therapy (ACPAT) or centres that are members of the Canine Hydrotherapy Association (CHA) or Institute of Canine Hydrotherapists (ICH).

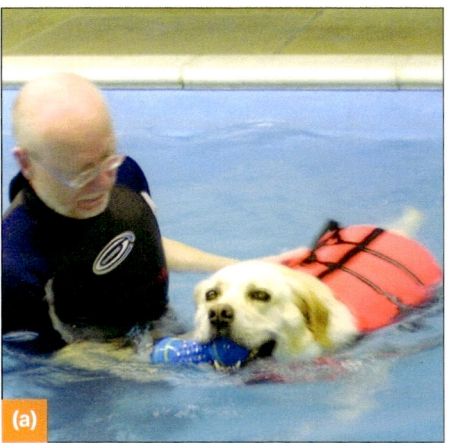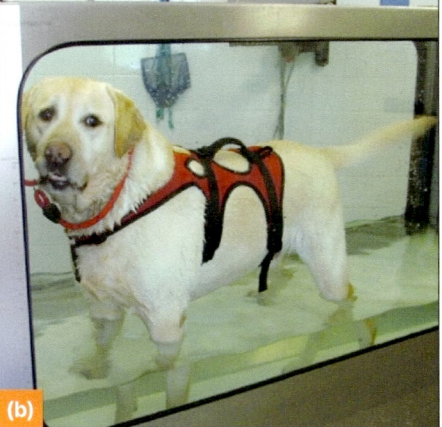

Figure 16.3: Hydrotherapy is most commonly undertaken in (a) a pool but can also take place on (b) an underwater treadmill.
(*Reproduced from BSAVA Manual of Canine and Feline Advanced Veterinary Nursing*)

Suitable diet choices

Suitable diets include:

- Adult maintenance diets
- 'Light' diets (modest caloric reduction only)
- Weight management diets (markedly calorie restricted)
- Alternative diet types (e.g. home-prepared cooked diets) (see Chapter 5).

Other management factors

Alleviating boredom and managing food-seeking behaviours

Many pets find periods of restricted activity difficult and frustrating, especially if they are used to a reliable routine of exercise. They do not understand that activity restriction is in their best interests in the long term. In addition, the use of analgesic drugs can increase frustration further because the pet is no longer in pain and may attempt to resume normal daily activities. This frustration can lead to undesirable behaviours (e.g. destruction and attention- or food-seeking). Owners should be advised that there are several ways to help their pet during this time. Encouraging pets to work for their food is a great way to challenge their mental ability, increase general activity and help manage some of the boredom or frustration-related behaviours that may be encountered.

- The daily food allocation can be divided into more than the usual two meals per day:
  - Feeding 4–6 smaller meals per day, each in a different way, can be more satisfying for the pet. Cats, in particular, prefer to consume food many times per day; up to 16 times per day has been reported (Thorne, 1982).
- Scatter feeding can be undertaken in the garden, on a patio or on an easily cleanable floor (e.g. kitchen floor).
- Homemade toys such as ice cube trays or toilet roll tube towers can be used (Figure 16.4a). Interactions must be supervised by the owner to prevent ingestion of any part of the toy.
- Commercially available puzzle toys and interactive feeding bowls can also be used (Figure 16.4b).
- The owner can use this opportunity to undertake training with their cat or to teach their dog a new command, reinforcing the pet–owner bond and giving the pet an outlet for any excess energy.
- Grooming can be an enjoyable pastime for a pet with restricted activity (without the need for additional food), as can gentle play with a favourite toy (provided this play can remain quiet and calm).

Communication with pet owners

Owners may initially be concerned about why their pet requires a period of restricted activity. Therefore, owners should be informed about the consequences if dietary control is not introduced. Convincing an owner of the importance of this can help ensure success.

At a time when an owner may be concerned that their pet might be suffering, they may be tempted to increase the number of treats and rewards given to make the pet feel better. Owners may also experience feelings of guilt associated with reduced activity and provide food as a substitute. Warning that there may be temptation to do this will hopefully bring it

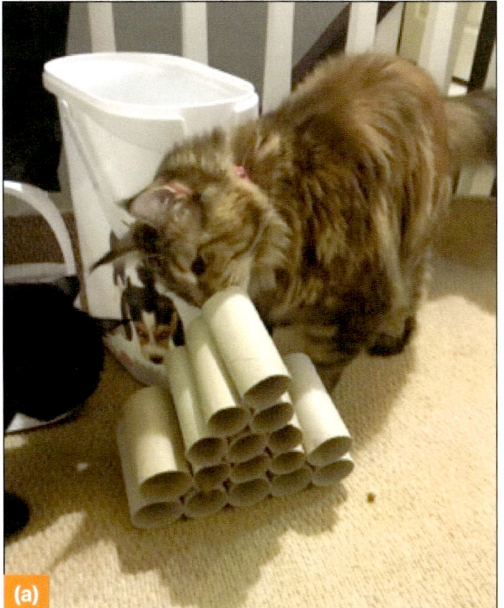

(a)

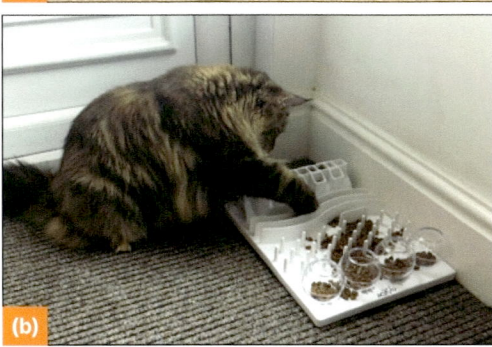

(b)

Figure 16.4: (a) Homemade toys and (b) interactive puzzle feeders can be useful for pets with restricted activity. (© Georgia Woods-Lee)

to the attention of the owner and prevent them from overfeeding. This must be coupled with strategies for what owners can do to help their pet throughout the period of activity restriction.

Should obesity already be present, this could be a good opportunity to discuss obesity care and weight reduction; however, it should be noted that initiation of the weight loss plan should only commence once the active phase of any illness has resolved. Especially in cases of long-term restricted activity, weight loss has been shown to have a huge impact on mobility. The improvements in mobility can be observed after just 6–9% weight loss (Marshall *et al.*, 2010). Many pet owners may feel that weight loss is not possible due to the low activity level. However, since weight loss relies on creating a negative energy balance (by food restriction and to a much lesser degree by increasing activity), although it may be slower during periods of restriction, it is still possible (see Chapter 15).

Conclusion

Periods of time where restricted activity is required can be challenging for both the pet and owner. It is important that the pet emerges from this period of restriction without having gained additional weight or developed undesirable behaviours. Some pets may always require some degree of activity restriction, so long-term solutions should be sought to ensure weight is controlled. With careful consideration about which foods should be provided and the methods of feeding, owners can help prevent weight gain, optimize the outcome and support their pet throughout this time.

References and further reading

Moore AH and Rudd S (2008) *BSAVA Manual of Canine and Feline Advanced Veterinary Nursing, 2nd edn.* BSAVA Publications, Gloucester

Keller E, Sagols E, Flanagan J, Biourge V and German AJ (2020) Use of reduced-energy content maintenance diets for modest weight reduction in overweight cats and dogs. *Research in Veterinary Science* **131**, 194–205

Marshall WG, Hazewinkel, Mullen D *et al.* (2010) The effect of weight loss on lameness in obese dogs with osteoarthritis. *Veterinary Research Communications* **34**, 241–253

Thorne CJ (1982) Feeding behaviour in the cat – recent advances. *Journal of Small Animal Practice* **23**, 555–562

Online extras

This chapter includes:

- **A client information leaflet that is available to download and print from the BSAVA Library**

Access via QR code or: bsavalibrary.com/nutrition_16

Diabetes mellitus

17

Diabetes mellitus (DM) is a chronic endocrine condition that affects both dogs and cats. It is a heterogeneous syndrome (Gilor *et al.*, 2016) which, left untreated, is detrimental to the pet. Two distinct types of DM have been recognized (Figure 17.1):

- Type I DM (insulin-dependent)
- Type II DM (non-insulin-dependent).

Type of diabetes mellitus	Cause	Management strategy
Type I Insulin-dependent	■ Destruction of the insulin-producing beta cells within the pancreas	■ Relies fully upon the provision of additional insulin ■ Consistent provision of nutrition and exercise
Type II Non-insulin-dependent	■ Tissue cell receptors are resistant to the effects of insulin, preventing glucose transportation ■ Closely associated with obesity and may result in hyperinsulinaemia ■ Most commonly seen in cats but has also been reported in dogs	■ Additional insulin frequently given to achieve good blood glucose control (but not in all cases) ■ Nutritional management ■ Weight loss programmes should be implemented if required

Figure 17.1: Causes of and management strategies for the types of diabetes mellitus seen in dogs and cats.

Under normal circumstances, when a dog or cat consumes food, the blood glucose concentration rises and stimulates the pancreas to produce insulin. The role of insulin is to act on cell receptors to allow glucose from the blood to enter the cells and be used as an energy source. When insufficient insulin is produced or there is resistance to its effects, cells are deprived of glucose, and hyperglycaemia and glycosuria develop (Fascetti and Delaney, 2023).

DM in dogs is typically associated with lack of insulin production (i.e. Type I DM). In contrast, cats tend to experience problems associated with resistance of the cell receptors to the effects of insulin, often because of obesity. This means that although insulin is being produced, it is not facilitating transportation of glucose from the blood into the cells (i.e. Type II DM). As resistance persists, the pancreas is stimulated to produce more insulin; however, this does not solve the problem but instead results in exhaustion of the beta cells, leading to an insulin-dependent type of DM similar to that observed in dogs.

The effect of nutrition

Nutrition plays a key role in the management strategies of both types of DM. It can help extend the lifespan of the pet and contribute to an improved quality of life.

- Type I DM – although dietary alterations cannot eliminate the requirement for exogenous insulin, they should help to improve overall glycaemic control.
- Type II DM – dietary management is an essential component of the overall strategy and, in some cases, can eventually eliminate the need for exogenous insulin.

Alongside insulin therapy, the ideal dietary solution for dogs involves provision of a stable and consistent routine by the owners. They require a diet with a low glycaemic index comprising complex carbohydrates that will release energy slowly throughout the day. For cats, the priority is feeding a diet that is low in carbohydrates and high in protein. If the cat has concurrent obesity, therapeutic weight reduction (see Chapter 15) should be considered, but only once the DM is stable. Cats can enter diabetic remission as a result of nutritional management, most notably following weight reduction.

Essential elements

Energy

The energy requirements of diabetic animals will differ. Weight loss is a common clinical sign, especially in poorly controlled cases. Weight gain may occur if there is a concurrent endocrinological condition (such as hyperadrenocorticism or hypothyroidism) or following successful stabilization of the DM. Obesity in both dogs and cats can predispose to DM. The relationship between obesity and DM in cats is well understood (Prahl *et al.*, 2007), with increasing degrees of obesity resulting in poorer insulin sensitivity (Appleton *et al.*, 2001). This relationship also exists in dogs but it is poorly understood. Energy restriction to facilitate therapeutic weight reduction can improve insulin sensitivity and therefore should be advised for any patient that is considered overweight or obese (German *et al.*, 2009) (see Chapter 15).

Water

Dogs and cats with DM may have increased water loss due to osmotic diuresis caused by glucosuria or ketoacidosis. Therefore, clean, fresh water should always be readily available and easily accessible. For senior pets and those with limited mobility, it may be helpful for the owner to provide multiple water sources around the home.

Protein

High protein diets are recommended because muscle wasting is common in individuals with poorly controlled DM. When insufficient protein is provided in the diet, proteins within the body are catabolized to produce an additional energy source to help meet the requirements of the pet (Freeman, 2018). This results in loss of muscle mass.

Fat

Abnormalities of lipid metabolism (e.g. hypercholesterolaemia and hypertriglyceridaemia) are common in dogs and cats with DM, as are systemic conditions such as pancreatitis. For these reasons, a fat-restricted diet should be provided (Fascetti and Delaney, 2012).

Carbohydrate

Diets containing simple carbohydrates should be avoided in favour of diets containing complex carbohydrates, as these help to improve glycaemic control (Fascetti *et al.*, 2023). In cats, high protein, low carbohydrate diets are beneficial for maintaining good glycaemic control.

Fibre

Although not traditionally considered to be an essential nutrient, large quantities of fibre are often fed to dogs with DM. Both soluble and insoluble fibre is thought to promote improved glycaemic control, increase satiety, reduce the calorie density of the diet, regulate gastrointestinal transit time and modulate nutrition absorption (Blaxter *et al.*, 1990; Nelson *et al.*, 2000).

Suitable diet choices

Dietetic foods (both wet and dry preparations) are available that have been formulated to assist with the management of DM. For cats that would benefit from a low carbohydrate diet, this may be more easily achieved using wet food. In addition, given that polyphagia is a common clinical sign when DM is initially diagnosed, the transition to an appropriate dietetic food is typically well received and completed without resistance in many patients.

Other management factors

Regular routine

A regular routine is required to achieve consistent glycaemic control, particularly in cases of Type I DM. The same type of food, brand and quantity should be fed at the same time each day. Diets with a fixed formula should be used (see Chapter 1). This helps ensure that there are no ingredient or composition changes, which might affect glycaemic control. Home-prepared diets (see Chapters 5 and 6) are usually not recommended for this reason. Any necessary dietary changes should be made gradually (e.g. over at least 7–10 days). In cats, it may be preferable to maintain their usual feeding regimen (if they are not obese or fed *ad libitum*) as transition from frequent feedings to twice a day meal provision may not be helpful.

Exercise

Consistency in all daily activities for dogs with DM is vital for good long-term glycaemic control. Given that exercise increases energy needs, varying the duration and intensity of walks can disrupt good control. Although this might be frustrating for owners, the importance of a consistent daily exercise regimen in terms of duration, intensity and time of day should be emphasized. It has been suggested that any alterations to the pattern or amount of physical activity should be gradually introduced to prevent significant changes in energy expenditure.

Preventing diabetes mellitus

Unfortunately, Type I DM cannot be prevented. In contrast, given that obesity is a known risk factor, the likelihood of Type II DM developing can be decreased by ensuring that dogs and cats maintain an ideal body condition. Dietetic food for therapeutic weight loss should be considered for pets that become overweight or obese. It should be noted that the incidence of Type II DM in cats increases with age (Sparkes *et al.*, 2015). Owners should be provided with information about the clinical signs of and risk factors for DM.

Communication with pet owners

Providing care for a pet with DM, particularly if the owner is required to administer insulin injections, is no small undertaking. Understandably, owners may initially feel daunted and uncertain whilst they learn about the disease and how to provide the correct medical management and appropriate diet. Veterinary surgeons (veterinarians) and veterinary nurses are well placed to provide support and reassurance to the owner. This may initially include demonstrations on how to administer insulin to their pet (Figure 17.2), how to store the insulin and guidance as to what clinical signs to monitor their pet for. Regular ongoing diabetic checks at the clinic allow the veterinary team to identify any complications arising from the management strategy and to take swift action to resolve them. The use of a daily diary may be helpful for the long-term management of DM. Information recorded in the diary may be vital should glycaemic control become poor or erratic. The diary should be reviewed on a regular basis and recommendations for action or appropriate advice given each time.

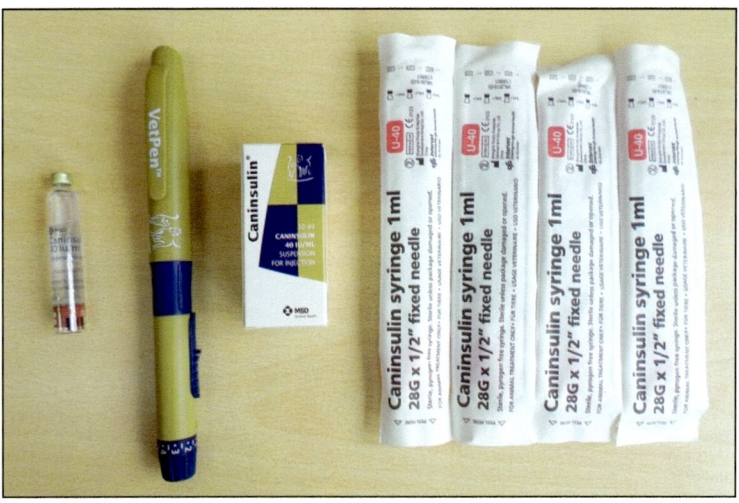

Figure 17.2: Caninsulin is one of the two types of insulin authorized for use in dogs. Caninsulin is available in two formulations: the VetPen and a suspension for injection with insulin syringes.
(Reproduced from the *BSAVA Manual of Canine and Feline Endocrinology*).

Conclusion

Nutrition plays a key role in the management of DM cases. It can help to maintain glycaemic control and improve the quality of life of the patient. In cases of Type II DM, appropriate nutrition can also help to induce clinical remission.

References and further reading

Appleton D, Rand J and Sunvold G (2001) Insulin sensitivity decreases with obesity, and lean cats with low insulin sensitivity are at greatest risk of glucose intolerance with weight gain. *Journal of Feline Medicine and Surgery* **3**, 211–228

Blaxter AC, Cripps PJ and Gruffydd-Jones TJ (1990) Dietary fibre and post prandial hyperglycaemia in normal and diabetic dogs. *Journal of Small Animal Practice* **31**, 229–233

Fascetti AJ and Delaney SJ (2012) *Applied Veterinary Clinical Nutrition*. John Wiley & Sons Ltd, Philadelphia

Fascetti AJ and Delaney SJ (2023) Nutritional management of endocrine diseases. In: *Applied Veterinary Clinical Nutrition*, ed. AJ Fascetti et al., pp. 441–448. Wiley Blackwell, Philadelphia

Fettman MJ, Stanton CA, Banks LL *et al.* (1998) Effects of weight gain and loss on metabolic rate, glucose tolerance, and serum lipids in domestic cats. *Research in Veterinary Science* **64**, 11–16

Freeman LM (2018) Cachexia and sarcopenia in companion animals: an under-utilized natural animal model of human disease. *JCSM Rapid Communications* **1**, 1–17

German AJ, Hervera M, Hunter L *et al.* (2009) Improvement in insulin resistance and reduction in plasma inflammatory adipokines after weight loss in obese dogs. *Domestic Animal Endocrinology* **37**, 214–226

Gilor C, Niessen SJM, Furrow E and DiBartola SP (2016) What's in a name? Classification of diabetes mellitus in veterinary medicine and why it matters. *Journal of Veterinary Internal Medicine* **30**, 927–940

Gostelow R, Forcada Y, Graves T *et al.* (2014) Systematic review of feline diabetic remission: separating fact from opinion. *Veterinary Journal* **202(2)**, 208–221

Gould D and McLellan GJ (2014) *BSAVA Manual of Canine and Feline Ophthalmology, 3rd edn*. BSAVA Publications, Gloucester

Holste LC, Nelson RW, Feldman EC and Bottoms GD (1989) Effect of dry, soft moist, and canned dog foods on postprandial blood glucose and insulin concentrations in healthy dogs. *American Journal of Veterinary Research* **50**, 984–989

Laflamme DP, Backus RC, Forrester SD and Hoenig M (2022) Evidence does not support the controversy regarding carbohydrates in feline diets. *Journal of the American Veterinary Medical Association* **260**, 506–513

Mooney CT, Peterson ME and Shiel RE (2023) *BSAVA Manual of Canine and Feline Endocrinology, 5th edn*. BSAVA Publications, Gloucester

Nelson RW, Scott-Moncrieff JC, Feldman EC *et al.* (2000) Effect of dietary insoluble fiber on control of glycemia in cats with naturally acquired diabetes mellitus. *Journal of the American Veterinary Medical Association* **216**, 1082–1088

Prahl A, Guptill L, Glickman NW, Tetrick M and Glickman LT (2007) Time trends and risk factors for diabetes mellitus in cats presented to veterinary teaching hospitals. *Journal of Feline Medicine and Surgery* **9**, 351–358

Sparkes AH, Cannon M, Church D *et al.* (2015) ISFM consensus guidelines on the practical management of diabetes mellitus in cats. *Journal of Feline Medicine and Surgery* **17**, 235–250

Zicker SC, Nelson RW, Kirk CA and Wedekind KJ (2010) Endocrine disorders. In: *Small Animal Clinical Nutrition* ed. MS Hand et al., pp. 415–427. Mark Morris Institute, Kansas

Online extras

This chapter includes:

● **A client information leaflet that is available to download and print from the BSAVA Library**

Access via QR code or: bsavalibrary.com/nutrition_17

Acute gastroenteritis

18

Gastroenteritis is a general term that describes dysfunction of the gastrointestinal (GI) tract and may present as acute (short term) or chronic (long term). Acute gastroenteritis refers to a digestive disturbance with a sudden onset and a short duration and is one of the most common reasons that cats and dogs are presented to a veterinary practice (O'Neill *et al.*, 2021). The diagnosis is typically based on signalment, presenting clinical signs (including pattern and severity), medical history and dietary history. In some cases, diagnostic tests such as biochemistry, haematology, faecal examination, endoscopy, radiography and ultrasonography are required to determine the cause. There are many causes of acute gastroenteritis (Figure 18.1). However, no matter the cause, the priority for management is to prevent nutritional deficiencies and restore normal function. In some cases, dietary modification alone is the sole management strategy.

Cause	Examples
Diet	Dietary indiscretion Rapid change of diet Hairballs (cats only) Food intolerance Adverse reactions to food (see Chapter 14)
Ingestion of a toxin or poisonous substance	Chocolate Xylitol (sweetener) Raisins or grapes Mouldy food
Drug induced	Antibiotics Non-steroidal anti-inflammatory drugs Chemotherapy drugs
Infectious	Bacterial agents Parasitic agents Viral agents (including parvovirus)
Systemic diseases	Pancreatitis Diabetic ketoacidosis Kidney disease (see Chapter 19) Hypoadrenocorticism (Addison's disease) Pyometra Liver disease (see Chapter 21)

Figure 18.1: Causes of acute gastroenteritis (continues). ▶

Cause	Examples
Inflammatory	Acute enteropathy (intestinal disease) Gastric ulcers
Obstruction	Foreign body Intussusception

Figure 18.1: (continued) Causes of acute gastroenteritis.

Faecal examination

The owner should be asked about the colour, smell, frequency, consistency and relationship of timing to feeding of any faecal output. It may also be useful to ask the owner to photograph the faeces or collect a sample for examination. This can help determine the location of disturbance within the GI tract.

- If the diarrhoea is caused by a problem in the small intestine, it is usually watery and the colour may be changed appearing more yellow than brown.
- If the diarrhoea is caused by a problem in the large intestine, there can be fresh blood and mucus. The act of defecation may also be accompanied by straining.
- Diarrhoea may be haemorrhagic and appear tarry black (digested blood) or bright red (fresh blood).

This highlights the importance of being aware of what constitutes a normal faecal output, not only in general terms, but also for the individual patient. Faecal scoring charts (Figure 18.2) can be very useful to facilitate this conversation with the pet owner. In addition, the scoring charts can be used to monitor faecal consistency over time.

The effect of nutrition

Nutrition plays a key role in the management strategy of acute gastroenteritis in both dogs and cats. Dietary adaptations help to assist recovery and prevent recurrence.

Essential elements

Energy

By feeding energy dense foods, energy requirements can be met with smaller meals compared with standard maintenance diets. This approach is particularly useful in cases of partial anorexia where only small volumes of food are being consumed. Given that these foods can have a high fat content, this should be taken into consideration to ensure that the diet is appropriate for the condition of the pet. As high fat diets can exacerbate diarrhoea, a gradual dietary transition should be undertaken to avoid this (see Chapter 2).

Protein

Protein-rich foods such as chicken, fish and scrambled egg are often fed with a carbohydrate source such as rice during episodes of acute gastroenteritis. Whilst acceptable for a short period of time (2–3 days maximum), such a diet should not be fed long term as it will not meet all the essential nutrient requirements.

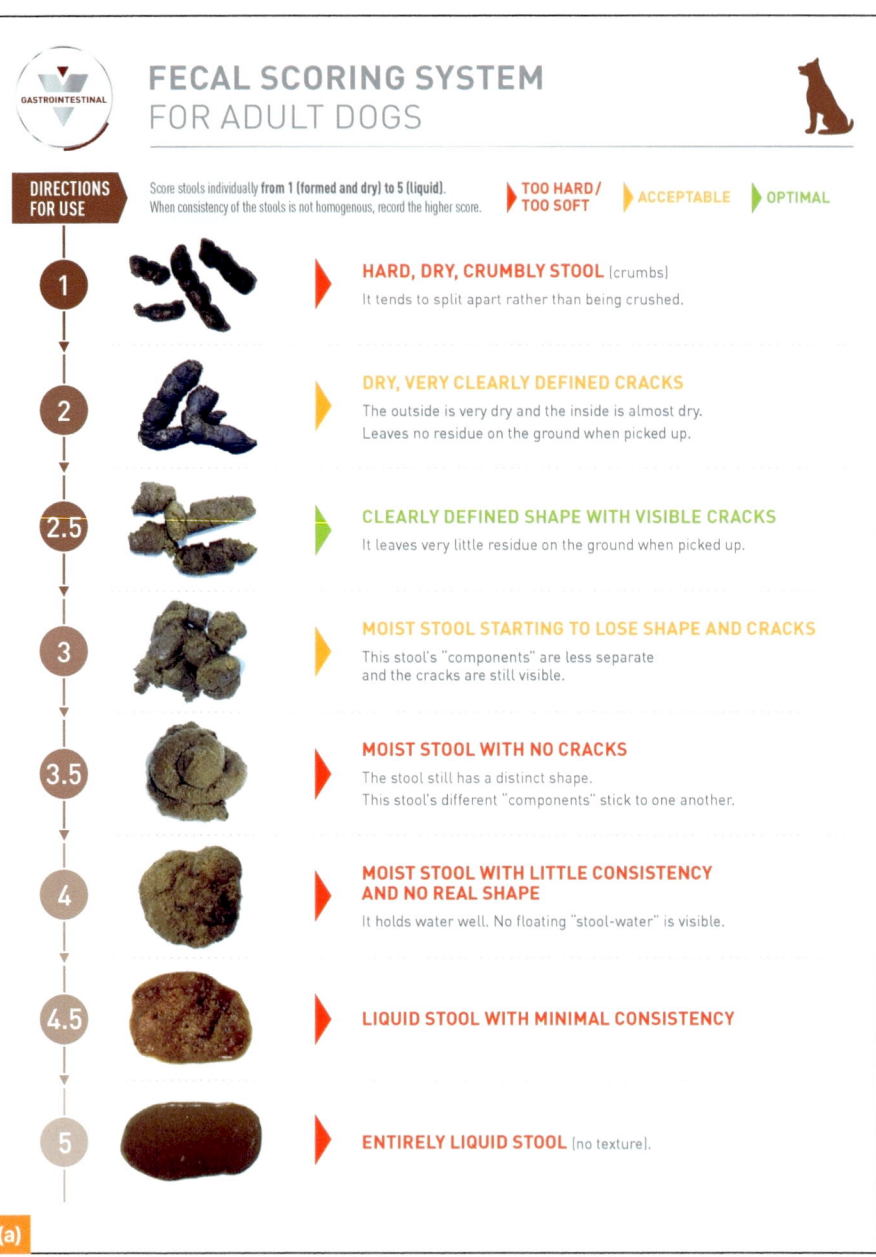

FECAL SCORING SYSTEM
FOR ADULT DOGS

DIRECTIONS FOR USE

Score stools individually **from 1 (formed and dry) to 5 (liquid)**.
When consistency of the stools is not homogenous, record the higher score.

▶ **TOO HARD / TOO SOFT**   ▶ **ACCEPTABLE**   ▶ **OPTIMAL**

1 — **HARD, DRY, CRUMBLY STOOL** (crumbs)
It tends to split apart rather than being crushed.

2 — **DRY, VERY CLEARLY DEFINED CRACKS**
The outside is very dry and the inside is almost dry.
Leaves no residue on the ground when picked up.

2.5 — **CLEARLY DEFINED SHAPE WITH VISIBLE CRACKS**
It leaves very little residue on the ground when picked up.

3 — **MOIST STOOL STARTING TO LOSE SHAPE AND CRACKS**
This stool's "components" are less separate
and the cracks are still visible.

3.5 — **MOIST STOOL WITH NO CRACKS**
The stool still has a distinct shape.
This stool's different "components" stick to one another.

4 — **MOIST STOOL WITH LITTLE CONSISTENCY AND NO REAL SHAPE**
It holds water well. No floating "stool-water" is visible.

4.5 — **LIQUID STOOL WITH MINIMAL CONSISTENCY**

5 — **ENTIRELY LIQUID STOOL** (no texture).

(a)

Figure 18.2: Faecal scoring charts for (a) dogs and (b) cats. (continues)
(© ROYAL CANIN® SAS 2025 used with permission).

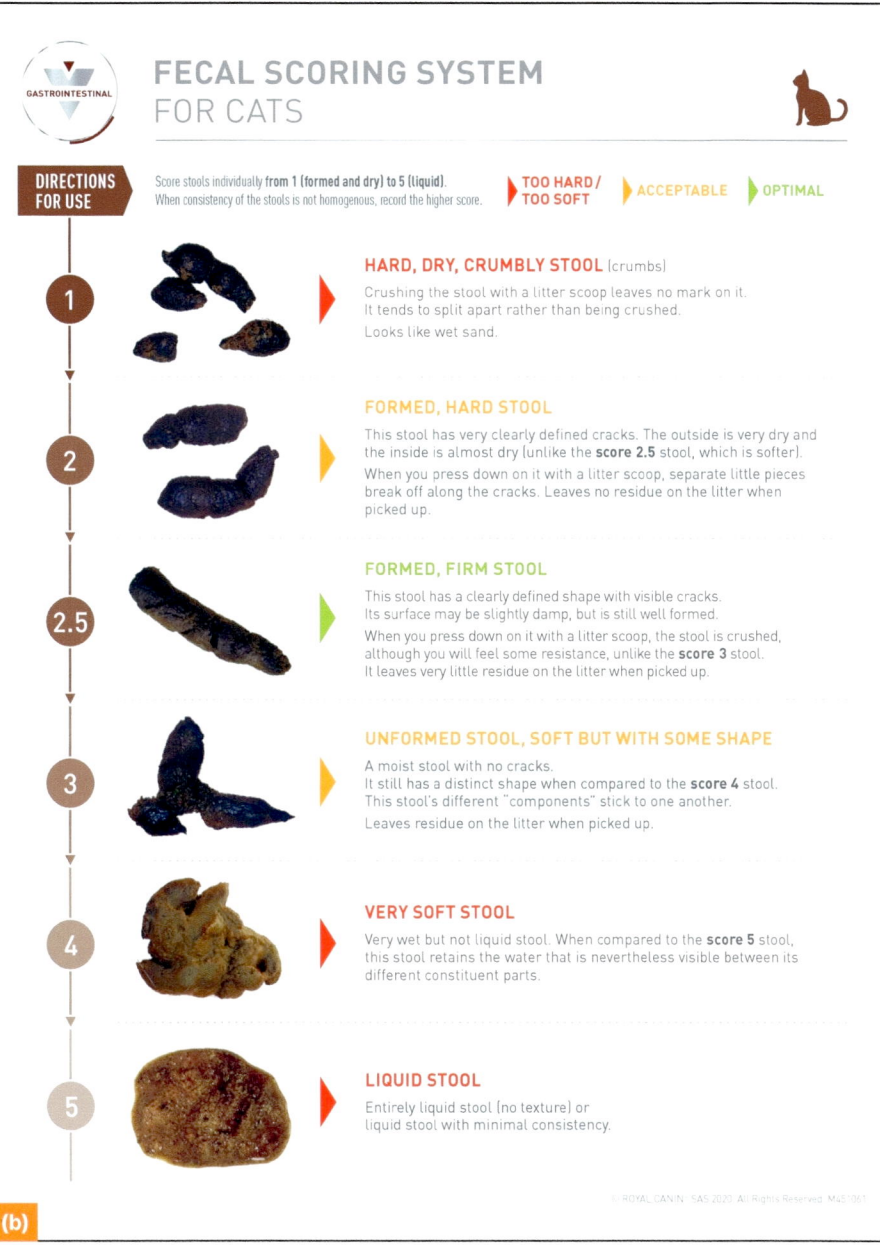

Figure 18.2: (continued) Faecal scoring charts for (a) dogs and (b) cats.
(© ROYAL CANIN® SAS 2025 used with permission).

Prebiotics

Prebiotics are non-digestible dietary carbohydrates such as fibre and starch. They are converted into short-chain fatty acids by the bacteria in the GI tract, which are then used as an energy source by the colonocytes. The inclusion of prebiotics in the diet, therefore, helps to improve GI tract health, improve digestion and inhibit pathogenic bacterial growth. However, in cases of acute diarrhoea, prebiotics have little or no clinical effect and the inclusion of the additional fibre could reduce the digestibility of the food provided (Scahill *et al.*, 2024).

Probiotics

Probiotics are live bacterial organisms that help normalize the microbiome of the GI tract and reduce GI disturbance (Kelley *et al.*, 2009). The use of probiotics is of some (although limited) benefit to patients with acute gastroenteritis (Jugan *et al.*, 2017) and may therefore be a useful addition to other dietary adaptations. As probiotics are not tightly regulated, choosing a commercial product that has undergone suitable trials for efficacy in acute diarrhoea cases and has sufficient quality control procedures is essential (Rallis *et al.*, 2016).

Vitamins

Folate and cobalamin are both associated with GI tract health. In cases of chronic diarrhoea (but not usually acute diarrhoea cases unless there is a pre-existing disease) the dysfunction of the GI tract can result in deficiencies.

Suitable diet choices

Purpose-formulated dietetic foods are commercially available that satisfy all nutritional requirements and are appropriate for patients with acute gastroenteritis; however, it may also be possible to use the patient's own diet provided it is complete and balanced, of good quality and no nutrient contained within it contraindicates its use (e.g. the fat content). Alternatively, home-prepared cooked diets can be fed (see Chapter 5) and, given that they are only required for a short period of time, there is no need for these diets to be formulated to be complete and balanced. Foods commonly used in home-prepared cooked diets include boiled chicken, fish or egg, often combined with boiled rice. In cases of adverse reactions to food, hydrolysed diets may also be suitable (see Chapter 14).

High digestibility

For any diet provided, the digestibility of the food should exceed 90% in order to prevent residual undigested food from entering the colon. Feeding a diet that is marketed as highly digestible helps to ensure optimal absorption of proteins, fats and carbohydrates. Highly digestible diets can also improve faecal consistency (Nery *et al.*, 2010).

High palatability

Foods with an increased fat and protein content are more palatable. High fat diets can slow gastric emptying so should be used with caution in cases where this is a problem (e.g. chronic or recurrent pancreatitis, hyperlipidaemia). Highly palatable foods are required to encourage voluntary food consumption.

Other management factors

There are two options for managing cases of acute gastroenteritis: a period of food withholding or so-called 'feeding through' where food continues to be provided.

Withholding food

With this approach, food is withheld for a short period of time (typically 12–24 hours) on the basis that allowing the animal to eat and drink as normal might exacerbate the clinical signs. This approach is particularly indicated for those animals that are vomiting, in conjunction with the use of antiemetic medication. Withholding food for more than 24 hours is rarely required. After this period of time, small amounts of food should be reintroduced; typically either a highly digestible commercially available dietetic diet (see Chapter 3) or home-prepared cooked diet (see Chapter 5).

> Short periods of withholding food are unlikely to be detrimental; withholding of food is not advisable for kittens and puppies with acute gastroenteritis (see Chapter 10).

Feeding through

With this approach, food continues to be offered either by mouth (mild cases can be managed by the owner at home) or via a feeding tube. Several studies have shown the benefits of early enteral feeding (Qin *et al.*, 2002; Mohr *et al.*, 2003; Chen *et al.*, 2004; Will *et al.*, 2005; Kawasaki *et al.*, 2009; Mansfield *et al.*, 2011; Liu *et al.*, 2012; Harris *et al.*, 2017; Hoffberg and Koenigshof, 2017; Wallace *et al.*, 2024). For cases managed at home, the frequency and type of food provided may need to be altered (e.g. increased frequency of meal provision with a highly digestible diet).

> There is little evidence of difference in efficacy for resting the GI tract *versus* the feeding through approach (Remillard, 2002). One exception is for cases of acute parvovirus enteritis in puppies, where improved outcomes are seen with early enteral nutrition using naso-oesophageal tube feeding (see Chapter 13).

Transitioning back to the previous diet

Once the clinical signs of acute gastroenteritis have ceased and faecal consistency has returned to normal, the dog or cat can gradually be transitioned back to their normal food, usually over at least 3–4 days (see Chapter 2).

Preventing acute gastroenteritis

The following factors should be considered to help prevent future episodes of acute gastroenteritis:

- Remove access to food waste bins to prevent scavenging and ingestion of toxins
- Prevent scavenging behaviours when out on walks
- Secure toxic or poisonous substances in an area of the home that the pet is unable to access
- Slowly transition all pets from one food to another if a change of diet is required

- Trial a different long-term diet (e.g. hydrolysed or novel protein diets; see Chapter 8)
- Investigate alternative drugs when one causes a gastrointestinal disturbance
- Continue management of any ongoing disease.

Communication with pet owners

Owners of pets with acute gastroenteritis may be distressed, especially if they have to deal with the animal vomiting and defecating within the house; in addition, the presence of blood within the vomitus or faeces can be alarming. Owners should be reassured that, in most cases, clinical signs will improve relatively quickly and the presence of a small amount of blood in the vomitus or faeces is unlikely to be the result of a serious condition. It is sensible to discuss with the owner where their pet should be housed (e.g. ideally in a comfortable location that is easy to keep clean). For long-haired dog and cat breeds, basic hygiene techniques (e.g. shaving hair around the anus, from the tail base and from the hindlimbs) can help to keep the pet clean until clinical signs resolve.

Conclusion

Nutrition plays a key role in the management of acute gastroenteritis cases. There is also some evidence that probiotics may lead to a more rapid resolution of clinical signs. Pet owners will often require support to manage any unexpected episodes of vomiting or soiling in the house.

References and further reading

Chen J, Wang XP, Liu P *et al.* (2004) Effects of continuous early enteral nutrition on the gut barrier function in dogs with acute necrotizing pancreatitis. *Zhonghua Yi Xue Za Zhi* **84(20)**, 1726–1731

Harris JP, Parnell NK, Griffith EH and Saker KE (2017) Retrospective evaluation of the impact of early enteral nutrition on clinical outcomes in dogs with pancreatitis: 34 cases (2010–2013) *Journal of Veterinary Emergency and Critical Care (San Antonio)* **27(4)**, 425–433

Hoffberg JE and Koenigshof A (2017) Evaluation of the safety of early compared to late enteral nutrition in canine septic peritonitis. *Journal of the American Animal Hospital Association* **52(2)**, 90–95

Jugan MC, Rudinsky AJ, Parker VJ and Gilor C (2017) Use of probiotics in small animal veterinary medicine. *Journal of the American Veterinary Medical Association* **250**, 519–528

Kawasaki N, Suzuki Y, Nakayoshi T *et al.* (2009) Early postoperative enteral nutrition is useful for recovering gastrointestinal motility and maintaining the nutritional status. *Surgery Today* **39(3)**, 225–230

Kelley RL, Minikhiem D, Kiely B *et al.* (2009) Clinical benefits of probiotic canine-derived *Bifidobacterium animalis* strain AHC7 in dogs with acute idiopathic diarrhea. *Veterinary Therapeutics* **10**, 121–130

Liu DT, Brown DC and Silverstein DC (2012) Early nutritional support is associated with decreased length of hospitalization in dogs with septic peritonitis: A retrospective study of 45 cases (2000–2009). *Journal of Veterinary Emergency and Critical Care (San Antonio)* **22(4)**, 453–459

Mansfield CS, James FE, Steiner JM, Suchodolski JS, Robertson ID and Hosgood G (2011) A pilot study to assess tolerability of early enteral nutrition via esophagostomy tube feeding in dogs with severe acute pancreatitis. *Journal of Veterinary Internal Medicine* **25(3)**, 419–425

Mazzaferro EM (2020) Update on canine parvoviral enteritis. *Veterinary Clinics of North America: Small Animal Practice* **50**, 1307–1325

Mohr AJ, Leisewitz AL, Jacobson LS, Steiner JM, Ruaux CG and Williams DA (2003) Effect of early enteral nutrition on intestinal permeability, intestinal protein loss, and outcome in dogs with severe parvoviral enteritis. *Journal of Veterinary Internal Medicine* **17(6)**, 791–798

Nery J, Biourge V, Tournier C *et al.* (2010) Influence of dietary protein content and source on fecal quality, electrolyte concentrations, and osmolarity, and digestibility in dogs differing in body size. *Journal of Animal Sciences* **88**, 159–169

O'Neill DG, James H, Brodbelt DC, Church DB and Pegram C (2021) Prevalence of commonly diagnosed disorders in UK dogs under primary veterinary care: results and applications. *BMC Veterinary Research* **17**, 1–15

Qin HL, Su ZD, Gao Q and Lin QT (2002) Early intrajejunal nutrition: bacterial translocation and gut barrier function of severe acute pancreatitis in dogs. *Hepatobiliary and Pancreatitis Diseases International* **1(1)**, 150–154

Rallis TS, Pardali D, Adamama-Moraitou KK and Kavarnos I (2016) Effect of Enterococcus faecium SF68®(Fortiflora®) administration in dogs with antibiotic responsive or small intestinal bacterial over-growth diarrhoea. *Hellenic Journal of Companion Animal Medicine* **5(2)**, 8–16

Remillard RL (2002) Nutritional support in critical care patients *Veterinary Clinics of North America: Small Animal Practice* **32**, 1145–1164

Scahill K, Jessen LR, Prior C *et al.* (2024) Efficacy of antimicrobial and nutraceutical treatment for canine acute diarrhoea: A systematic review and meta-analysis for European Network for Optimization of Antimicrobial Therapy (ENOVAT) guidelines. *The Veterinary Journal* **303**, 106054

Wallace OP, Jablonski SA, Thomas JS, Bock JH 3rd and Langlois DK (2024) Association of time to start of enteral nutrition and outcome in cats with hepatic lipidosis. *Journal of Veterinary Internal Medicine* **38(6)**, 3144–3152

Will K, Nolte I and Zentek J (2005) Early enteral nutrition in young dogs suffering from haemorrhagic gastroenteritis. *Journal of Veterinary Medicine* **52(7)**, 371–376

Online extras

This chapter includes:

● **A client information leaflet that is available to download and print from the BSAVA Library**

Access via QR code or: bsavalibrary.com/nutrition_18

Kidney disease

19

Kidney disease is divided into two categories:

- Acute kidney injury (AKI)
- Chronic kidney disease (CKD).

AKI is caused by an initial insult such as trauma, blockage, infection, toxin, neoplasia or ischaemia, or can occur when a patient with CKD experiences an exacerbating factor such as pyometra, dehydration or pancreatitis. Dietary management for these cases is of a supportive nature and dietetic food formulated for renal disease may only be needed if renal impairment persists. The most important factor for managing AKI is swift and aggressive intravenous fluid therapy.

CKD is a common progressive disease which can be differentiated from AKI by the clinical findings and history, laboratory test results and, in some cases, ultrasonography and histology results (Segev, 2025). In both dogs and cats, it is a primary cause of mortality and a reduced quality of life. Normal renal function relies upon functional nephrons to filter waste products from the blood and to excrete them via the urine. In the presence of CKD, there is an increasing loss of functional nephrons, which reduces the efficiency of excretion and causes a build-up of nitrogenous waste products and other uraemic toxins in the blood. This eventually results in a uraemic syndrome that affects multiple organs (Nigam and Bush, 2019).

The kidneys have a large functional reserve, which means that clinical signs of CKD are evident only in the later stages of the disease when 75–80% loss of functional nephrons has occurred. This highlights the need for regular screening of at-risk patients (e.g. senior pets) or prior to the administration of drugs that may affect kidney function. The International Renal Interest Society (IRIS) has developed a staging system for CKD based on blood creatinine and symmetric dimethylarginine (SDMA) concentrations (Figure 19.1). This staging system is a useful tool in the diagnosis and management of patients with CKD. An AKI grading system is also avaialble (Cowgill, 2016).

The effect of nutrition

There is no cure for CKD but with the appropriate nutritional adaptations, life expectancy and quality of life can be significantly increased (Elliott et al., 2000). A primary goal of dietary management is to reduce the intake of phosphorus. Nutritional adaptations are required when the serum phosphorus concentration is >1.5 mmol/l (IRIS recommendation) and the urine protein:creatinine ratio is increased. Other aims of dietary management include decreasing nitrogenous waste products and uraemic toxins, preserving remaining nephron function and reducing the rate of further nephron damage.

IRIS classification	Blood creatinine concentration (µmol/l)		Blood creatinine concentration (mg/dl)		Symmetric dimethylarginine concentration (µg/dl)	
	Cats	Dogs	Cats	Dogs	Cats	Dogs
Stage 1	<140	<125	<1.6	<1.4	<18	<18
Stage 2	140–250	125–250	1.6–2.8	1.4–2.8	18–25	18–35
Stage 3	251–440	251–440	2.9–5	2.9–5	26–38	36–54
Stage 4	>440	>440	>38	>5	>38	>54

Figure 19.1: International Renal Interest Society (IRIS) staging system for chronic kidney disease in dogs and cats.

Essential elements

Water

Polydipsia and polyurea are typically seen in pets with CKD. Increasing water intake will help to maintain hydration and should be encouraged. This can be achieved by:

- Feeding wet food – wet food typically contains 80% water compared with dry food which typically contains 8–10% water
- Adding water to food
- Ensuring that there are multiple water sources available – bowls should be placed on all floors that the pet has access to. This is especially important for senior pets as their mobility may be limited
- Offering different water delivery systems – providing a running water source (e.g. water fountain) and different types of bowl may be helpful, particularly in cats (Pachel and Neilson, 2010; Bartges, 2012). Many cats appear to prefer drinking from shallow ceramic or Pyrex® bowls rather than plastic or deep metal bowls. Water should be replaced and bowls cleaned frequently
- Using hydration supplements – nutritional products have been developed that can be included in a feeding regimen (e.g. PRO PLAN® HC Hydra Care).

Monitoring water intake is important in these cases because any increase might be indicative of disease progression or concurrent disorders. A measuring jug can be used to measure the volume of water provided to the pet and how much is left at the end of the day in order to calculate the amount drunk over a set time period. Routine recording of this information can be used to track trends and flag any significant changes. In addition, developments in technology mean that water intake can also now be measured accurately using a special bowl (e.g. Felaqua bowls by Sure Petcare®). These bowls measure the volume and frequency of water intake each day and send the data to the associated smart phone application. This application collates the information so that the owner can quickly and easily observe how much their pet has drunk each day. Where increased water intake and urine output is noted, further testing is advised as adjustments to treatment may be required.

Phosphorus

Serum phosphorus and calcium concentrations should be closely monitored. In pets with CKD, excretion of phosphorus by the kidneys is significantly impaired. This can lead to an increase in serum phosphorus concentration. Persistently increased serum phosphorus concentrations can lead to further renal damage and greater impairment of excretion. Although no commercial test is currently available, the type of phosphorus present (i.e. organic or inorganic) may be relevant, as the bioavailability of the two types differ. In addition, given that phosphorus and calcium homeostasis are closely linked, any increase in the serum phosphorus concentration causes a decrease in the serum calcium concentration. This results in stimulation of the parathyroid gland to produce parathyroid hormone, which in turn initiates demineralization of bone in an attempt to increase the serum calcium concentration. This condition is known as secondary renal hyperparathyroidism (Figure 19.2) or mineral bone disease and can lead to brittle bones and an increased risk of fractures.

For these reasons, dietary phosphorus should be restricted in pets with CKD. The aim is to maintain a serum phosphorus concentration >0.9 mmol/l but <1.5 mmol/l. This can be achieved using specifically formulated dietetic foods for kidney disease. In cases where the pet does not accept the dietetic food, the owner is unwilling to use the dietetic food, transition to the dietic food has failed despite all efforts or the serum phosphorus concentration remains elevated despite the use of a renal diet, then phosphate binders may be used (Bartges, 2012). These should be added to the food and work by trapping the phosphorus upon ingestion. However, the overall effect of phosphate binders is less reliable than use of a dietetic food that has been specifically formulated to be low in phosphorus.

Calcium

Hypercalcaemia can be a complication in cats with CKD. Dietary factors, such as a very low phosphorus concentration and imbalances in the calcium:phosphorus (Ca:P) ratio, may cause or exacerbate the condition. Should hypercalcaemia occur, the management strategy for such cases includes dietary modifications, such as diets with 200 mg/ calcium/100 kcal and a Ca:P ratio less than 1.4:1 (Ehrlich et al., 2024), as well as regular monitoring for biochemical parameters (van den Broek et al., 2017).

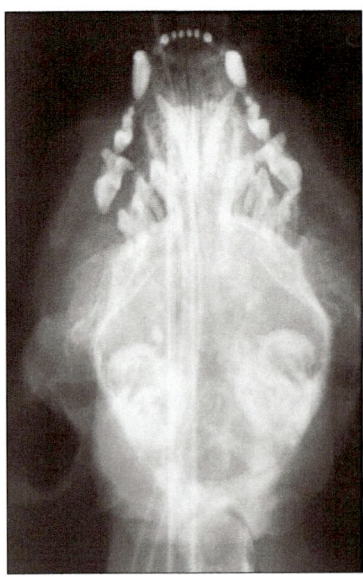

Figure 19.2: An osteopenic skull and the appearance of 'floating teeth' in a cat with renal secondary hyperparathyroidism.
(Reproduced from the *BSAVA Manual of Canine and Feline Musculoskeletal Disorders*)

Protein

Amino acids are metabolized by the liver where they form part of the urea cycle, with the resulting urea and other nitrogenous waste products subsequently being excreted by the kidneys. In pets with CKD, excretory function is decreased because of a loss of working nephrons. This results in the accumulation of nitrogenous waste, which becomes toxic, particularly during the later stages of CKD where it exacerbates the consequences of uraemic syndrome. The build up of nitrogenous waste products in the blood can be used as biomarkers for the presence of disease. Protein restriction can help limit the accumulation of nitrogenous waste but, since amino acids are essential nutrients, care must be taken to ensure that all nutritional requirements are met. This can be achieved by feeding proteins of high quality and high digestibility, so that all amino acid requirements are met from a smaller quantity of protein. Cats have a greater requirement for protein in their diet compared with dogs. This requirement is usually met by including proteins of animal origin (Ross *et al.*, 2006). Formulating these diets can be challenging, not least because animal-based protein products are also the main source of dietary phosphorus.

Potassium

Serum potassium concentrations should be closely monitored. Due to the increased water turnover associated with CKD, a considerable amount of potassium can be lost in the urine. Hypokalaemia can result in muscle weakness, lethargy, ventroflexion of the neck (cats) and appetite loss. It is advisable to replace the ongoing losses (Bartges, 2012); therefore, dietetic food formulated for patients with CKD contains higher concentrations of potassium for this purpose. However, it should be noted that some patients may become hyperkalaemic on renal diets. In these cases, a homemade diet may be required.

Sodium

Increased sodium intake may be damaging to the kidneys, so excessive amounts in the diet should be avoided (Bartges *et al.*, 1996).

Suitable diet choices

For patients with IRIS stage 1 CKD, current guidance suggests that diets formulated to have a lower phosphorus content than adult maintenance diets (e.g. specifically formulated dietetic foods for early renal care or senior diets with mildly restricted phosphorus) might be of benefit. Moreover, moderate phosphorus restriction may provide additional benefits for the long-term management of these cases (Hall *et al.*, 2019). For patients with IRIS stage 2 CKD and above, specifically formulated dietetic food with restricted phosphorus concentrations and moderate amounts of protein should be provided.

Other management factors

Transitioning to a new food

Since feeding the correct diet can increase life expectancy and the quality of life for pets with CKD, helping them to transition to the optimal diet is essential (see Chapter 2). The speed of the process depends on the individual and should never be rushed. In some cases, a small amount of a highly palatable food (e.g. chicken) may be useful to help ensure a successful food transition. The quantity used should not unbalance the diet and it should be gradually withdrawn upon completion of the transition. In some cases, successful transition to an appropriate food can take months (Quimby and Lunn, 2013; Quimby et al., 2020); owners must be directed appropriately and supported throughout this extended transition.

Treat management

Many pet foods and treats contain significant amounts of protein and phosphorus because these elements increase palatability. Given how important offering treats as a form of affection is, most owners will not accept the complete cessation of such behaviour. Therefore, alternative options such as courgette, broccoli and cauliflower could be suggested. An additional benefit of offering green watery vegetables as a treat option is the increase in water intake.

Supplements

The addition of eicosapentaenoic acids (EPAs) to the diet might prolong survival times for both dogs and cats with CKD (Brown et al., 2000; Plantinga et al., 2005). EPAs are derived from fish oils and are thought to help reduce inflammation (Brown et al., 2000). Some renal diets already contain sufficient quantities of EPAs; therefore, the ingredient information printed on the packaging of these diets should always be checked before the use of an EPA supplement, as excessive amounts could be detrimental.

Antioxidants

The loss of functional nephrons associated with CKD leads to oxidative stress; therefore, the addition of antioxidants to the diet might help combat the production of free radicals and slow progression of the disease (Brown, 2008). However, it is not clear which products are of most benefit, how they function and at what point they should be introduced to the diet. Further work, including clinical trials, is required before antioxidants can be recommended.

Misconceptions for feeding a patient with chronic kidney disease

Adult maintenance diets can be fed

For patients with IRIS stage 1 CKD and no proteinuria, feeding an adult maintenance diet may be possible in the short term but is not necessarily the best option. For long-term management, dietary changes may be required (Hall et al., 2019). For patients with IRIS stage 2 CKD and above, dietetic food with restricted phosphorus concentrations and moderate amounts of protein is recommended to avoid increasing the workload of the kidneys and accelerating disease progression.

Any diet type can be fed

Not all diet types are appropriate for the management of CKD. For example, the use of home-prepared cooked diets and raw meat-based diets should be carefully considered as they have been frequently shown to be unbalanced, with multiple nutritional deficiencies (Larsen et al., 2012).

- **Home-prepared cooked diets:** these diets can be formulated with the necessary restrictions; however, this should only ever be attempted or overseen by a person with a suitable qualification to avoid nutritional inadequacies (see Chapters 1 and 5).
- **Raw meat-based diets:** patients with CKD typically require a diet with restricted phosphorus content, which can be difficult to achieve with a raw diet (see Chapter 6).

Commercially manufactured foods contain preservatives that can cause disease

There is no evidence to substantiate the claim that commercially manufactured foods (especially in kibble form) contain preservatives that can cause CKD. Most cats and dogs fed commercially manufactured diets do not acquire CKD. Furthermore, cats and dogs fed alternative diets (e.g. raw meat-based diets or home-prepared cooked diets) still suffer from CKD. Therefore, food is unlikely to be a causal factor for disease. However, inorganic phosphorus salts, which are often added to processed pet food might be associated with disturbances of calcium and phosphorus homeostasis. Further work is required to determine the significance of these findings (Dobenecker *et al.*, 2021).

Feeding dry foods causes dehydration that can lead to renal damage

In a review of three published studies, there was no association between diet and the development of CKD (Hughes *et al.*, 2002; Greene *et al.*, 2014; McLeonard, 2017). However, dry diets might actually decrease the risk of developing CKD in cats (Piyarungsri and Pusoonthornthum, 2017). Further work is required in this area.

Communication with pet owners

It is important to help owners understand that, whilst CKD is not a disease that can be cured, its progression can be slowed and the quality of life of their pet can be improved. One of the most important ways this can be achieved is through dietary management. Owners have a huge role to play and their compliance with the dietary recommendations can help extend the life expectancy of their pet. In most cases, with support from the veterinary team, pet owners are able to make the necessary changes.

Conclusion

Nutrition plays a key role in the management of CKD cases. Although CKD is a progressive incurable disease, optimal nutritional management with the use of dietetic food can help prolong the life of the pet.

References and further reading

Arthurs G, Brown G and Pettitt R (2018) *BSAVA Manual of Canine and Feline Musculoskeletal Disorders, 2nd edn.* BSAVA Publications, Gloucester

Bartges JW (2012) Chronic kidney disease in dogs and cats. *Veterinary Clinics of North America: Small Animal Practice* **42**, 669–692

Bartges JW, Willis AM and Polzin DJ (1996) Hypertension and renal disease. *Veterinary Clinics*

of North America: Small Animal Practice **26**, 1331–1345

Brown SA (2008) Oxidative stress and chronic kidney disease. *Veterinary Clinics of North America: Small Animal Practice* **38**, 157–166

Brown SA, Brown CA, Crowell WA *et al.* (2000) Effects of dietary polyunsaturated fatty acid supplementation in early renal insufficiency in dogs. *Journal of Laboratory and Clinical Medicine* **135**, 275–286

Cowgill L (2016) Grading of acute kidney injury. Available from: www.iris-kidney.com/iris-guidelines-1 [Accessed on: 03/07/2025]

Dobenecker B, Reese S and Herbst S (2021) Effects of dietary phosphates from organic and inorganic sources on parameters of phosphorus homeostasis in healthy adult dogs. *PLoS One* **16**, e0246950

Ehrlich MR, Rudinsky AJ, Chew DJ and Parker VJ (2024) Ionized hypercalcemia can resolve with nutritional modification in cats with idiopathic hypercalcemia or chronic kidney disease. *Journal of Feline Medicine and Surgery* **24(2)**, 1098612X241229811

Elliott J, Rawlings JM, Markwell PJ and Barber PJ (2000) Survival of cats with naturally occurring chronic renal failure: effect of dietary management. *Journal of Small Animal Practice* **41**, 235–242

Greene JP, Lefebvre SL, Wang M *et al.* (2014) Risk factors associated with the development of chronic kidney disease in cats evaluated at primary care veterinary hospitals. *Journal of the American Veterinary Medical Association* **244**, 320–327

Hall JA, Fritsch DA, Jewell DE, Burris PA and Gross KL (2019) Cats with IRIS stage 1 and 2 chronic kidney disease maintain body weight and lean muscle mass when fed food having increased caloric density, and enhanced concentrations of carnitine and essential amino acids. *Veterinary Record* **184**, 190

Hughes KL, Slater MR, Geller S, Burkholder WJ and Fitzgerald C (2002) Diet and lifestyle variables as risk factors for chronic renal failure in pet cats. *Preventive Veterinary Medicine* **55**, 1–15

Larsen JA, Parks EM, Heinze CR and Fascetti AJ (2012) Evaluation of recipes for home-prepared diets for dogs and cats with chronic kidney disease. *Journal of the American Veterinary Medical Association* **240**, 532–538

Lefebvre S (2013) Clinical findings in cats and dogs with chronic kidney disease. *Veterinary Focus* **23**, 26–27

McLeonard CA (2017) Are adult cats fed on wet maintenance diets less at risk of developing chronic kidney disease compared to adult cats fed on dry maintenance diets? *Veterinary Evidence* **2(4)** DOI: 10.18849/ve.v2i4.130

Nigam SK and Bush KT (2019) Uraemic syndrome of chronic kidney disease: altered remote sensing and signalling. *Nature Reviews Nephrology* **15**, 301–316

Pachel C and Neilson J (2010) Comparison of feline water consumption between still and flowing water sources: a pilot study. *Journal of Veterinary Behaviour* **5**, 130–133

Piyarungsri K and Pusoonthornthum R (2017) Risk and protective factors for cats with naturally occurring chronic kidney disease. *Journal of Feline Medicine and Surgery* **19**, 358–363

Plantinga EA, Everts H, Kastelein AMC and Beynen AC (2005) Retrospective study of the survival of cats with acquired chronic renal insufficiency offered different commercial diets. *Veterinary Record* **157**, 185–187

Quimby J, Benson KK, Summers SC *et al.* (2020) Assessment of compounded transdermal mirtazapine as an appetite stimulant in cats with chronic kidney disease. *Journal of Feline Medicine and Surgery* **22(4)**, 376–383

Quimby J and Lunn KF (2013) Mirtazapine as an appetite stimulant and anti-emetic in cats with chronic kidney disease: a masked placebo-controlled crossover clinical trial. *Veterinary Journal* **197(3)**, 651–655

Ross SJ, Osborne CA, Kirk CA *et al.* (2006) Clinical evaluation of dietary modification for treatment of spontaneous chronic kidney disease in cats. *Journal of the American Veterinary Medical Association* **229**, 949–957

Segev G (2025) Differentiation between acute kidney injury and chronic kidney disease. Availabe from: www.iris-kidney.com/about [Accessed on: 03/07/2025]

van den Broek DHN, Chang YM, Elliott J and Jepson RE (2017) Chronic kidney disease in cats and the risk of total hypercalcemia. *Journal of Veterinary Internal Medicine* **31(2)**, 465–475

Online extras

This chapter includes:

- **A client information leaflet that is available to download and print from the BSAVA Library**

Access via QR code or: bsavalibrary.com/nutrition_19

Lower urinary tract disease | 20

The term lower urinary tract disease (LUTD) is used to describe diseases affecting the bladder and urethra. Although LUTD is seen in dogs, it occurs more commonly in cats. There are many possible causes of LUTD including urinary tract infection (UTI), urethral obstruction (more common in male than female pets), urinary crystal and urolith formation and feline interstitial cystitis (FIC). Obesity, decreased activity levels and multiple pets in the home have been associated with an increased risk of LUTD in cats. Feline interstitial cystitis is a type of feline lower urinary tract disease (FLUTD), which is the result of complex interactions between the adrenal glands, bladder, urethra and the neurological system, in conjunction with husbandry practices and the environment (Forrester and Towell, 2015). The condition occurs in both male and female cats, with neutered males at increased risk (He *et al.*, 2022). Typically, affected cats are between 1 and 10 years old (peak risk is 2–6 years of age), spend the majority of their time indoors, use litter trays exclusively and have a diet consisting of 75–100% dry food. Cats that have access to the outdoors can still be affected if they find the environment threatening.

The clinical signs associated with LUTD include pollakiuria (increased urination frequency), haematuria (the presence of blood in the urine), stranguria (difficulty passing urine) and periuria (urination in the home environment outside of the litter box for cats).

In healthy cats and dogs, the optimal pH for urine is approximately 6.0–7.5 (Chew *et al.*, 2010). When the pH consistently deviates from this range, depending on the minerals present in the urine, urinary crystals and uroliths may form (Figure 20.1).

Urinary crystal or urolith type	Urine pH	Mineral composition	Comments
Struvite (Figure 20.2a)	7 or above (alkaline)	■ Magnesium ■ Ammonium ■ Phosphate	■ Sterile crystals may be seen in healthy dogs and cats (no infectious agents present) – more common in cats ■ Associated with infection by urease-producing bacteria (e.g. *Staphylococcus* spp.) – more common in dogs (Teh, 2022) ■ Affects all breeds of dogs and cats (Klausner *et al.*, 1981; Palma *et al.*, 2009)

Figure 20.1: Types of urinary crystals and uroliths commonly encountered and the conditions required for their formation. (continues) (Data adapted from Minnesota Urolith Center). ▶

Urinary crystal or urolith type	Urine pH	Mineral composition	Comments
Calcium oxalate (Figure 20.2b)	6 or below (acidic)	■ Calcium (high concentration) ■ Oxalate (high concentration) ■ Hydroxyproline (high concentration, precursor to oxalate) ■ Magnesium (low concentration)	■ Factors affecting formation are not fully understood making this a difficult urolith to prevent ■ Crystals may be seen in healthy dogs and cats ■ Breeds frequently affected by uroliths include English Bulldogs (Saver *et al.*, 2021), French Bulldogs, Miniature Schnauzers (Kopecny *et al.*, 2021), Standard Poodles (Kopecny *et al.*, 2021) and Persian cats (Bartges *et al.*, 2016)
Cystine (Figure 20.2c)	6 or below (acidic)	■ Sodium	■ The accumulation of cystine may be caused by a hereditary defect that decreases transportation through the kidney, which is where cystine is normally removed from the urine ■ Breeds frequently affected include Dachshunds (Kovaříková *et al.*, 2021), English Bulldogs (Roe *et al.*, 2012), French Bulldogs and Staffordshire Bull Terriers
Urate (Figure 20.2d)	6 or below (acidic)	■ Purines	■ The accumulation of uric acid may be caused by a hereditary mutation of the *SLC2A9* gene or a portosystemic shunt. In both cases, transportation of uric acid to the liver (where it is degraded to allantonin) is decreased (Defarges *et al.*, 2020) ■ Breeds frequently affected include Dalmatians (Bartages *et al.*, 1999) and Yorkshire Terriers

Figure 20.1: (continued) Types of urinary crystals and uroliths commonly encountered and the conditions required for their formation.
(Data adapted from Minnesota Urolith Center).

The effect of nutrition

Nutrition is one component of the overall management strategy for LUTD. The environment within the urine can be influenced by nutrition (Finke and Litzenberger, 1992; Osbourne *et al.*, 2009); for example, some diets designed to affect the urine pH can help dissolve uroliths or decrease the risk of their formation in the future.

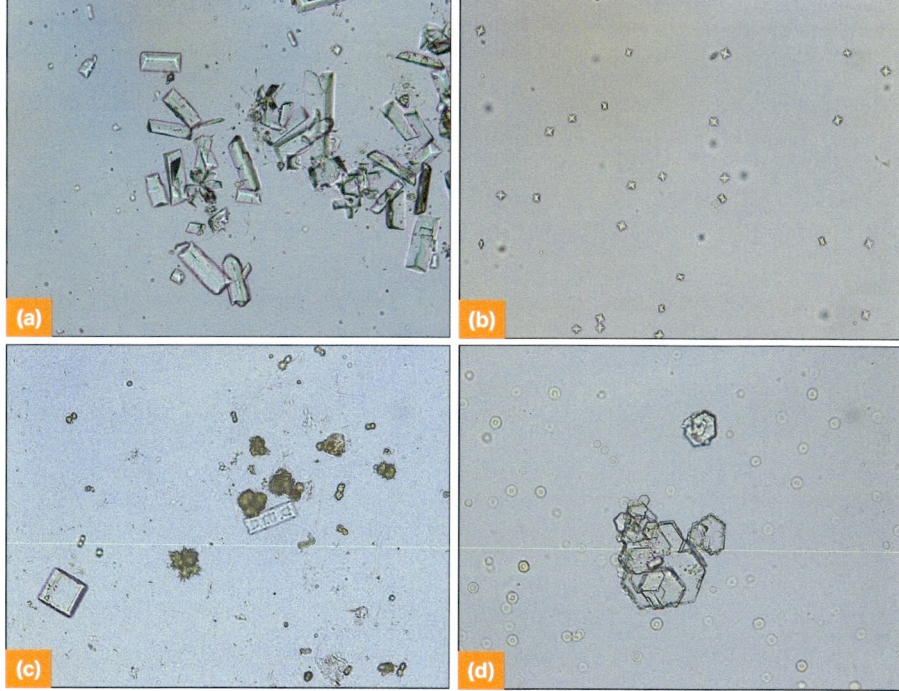

Figure 20.2: Urinary crystals: (a) struvite, (b) calcium oxalate, (c) cystine and (d) urate.
(Reproduced from *BSAVA Manual of Canine and Feline Clinical Pathology*)

Essential elements

Water

Any pet with LUTD should be encouraged to increase their water intake (Bartges and Corbee, 2023). This can be achieved by:

- Feeding wet food – wet food typically contains 80% water compared with dry food which typically contains 8–10% water
- Adding water to food
- Offering green watery vegetables (e.g. courgette) as treats
- Providing clean fresh water and using clean water bowls
- Changing the type of bowl provided – some dogs and cats may prefer to drink from a wide, shallow ceramic or Pyrex bowl®, rather than a plastic or deep metal bowl (Nowak, 2022)
- Providing a water fountain (Pachel and Neilson, 2010)
- For cats, it is important to ensure that water sources are in a different area to their food and litter tray (Ellis *et al.*, 2013)
- Hydration supplements are now available (e.g. PRO PLAN® HC Hydra Care; Zanghi *et al.*, 2018ab) that can be included in a feeding regimen
- Offering a homemade or a shop bought low-salt broth as an alternative to water.

> **Homemade chicken broth**
> 1. Boil a chicken breast in a pan of water until cooked. The chicken will impart flavour and aroma to the water. Do not add salt to the cooking water.
> 2. Once cooked, set chicken aside.
> 3. Allow the cooking liquid (broth) to cool before offering it to the pet in a suitable bowl or adding it to food.

Increasing water intake helps to prevent supersaturation of the urine. Supersaturation refers to a urinary environment where solutes (e.g. calcium, phosphate, cystine, oxalate) exceed their solubility limits and precipitate in the urine to form crystals and, eventually, uroliths. It is important, therefore, to ensure that the urine specific gravity (a measure of the degree of dilution of the urine) is kept below 1.020 in dogs and below 1.030 in cats.

Suitable diet choices

Dietetic foods (both wet and dry preparations) have been formulated to assist with the management of LUTD. The wet diets have an increased water content to help reduce the urine specific gravity (see above), may include omega-3 fatty acids, antioxidants, L-tryptophan or alpha-casozepine, and have variably decreased amounts of lithogenic minerals. Dietetic foods are particularly helpful in the management of urinary crystals and uroliths. The specific dietary adaptations required depend on the composition of the uroliths and are detailed in Figure 20.3.

Other management factors

Stress reduction

For cats with cystitis, stress is thought to be a compounding risk factor; therefore, methods for reducing environmental stress should be explored and implemented (Gülersoy et al., 2023). The American Association of Feline Practitioners (AAFP) and the International Society of Feline Medicine (ISFM) have published guidelines (including a client brochure) on multimodal environmental modification (MEMO), which can be used to make recommendations to owners about the ways they can help reduce stress for pets with FLUTD (Buffington et al., 2006; Ellis et al., 2013). In addition, nutraceuticals such as L-tryptophan or alpha-casozepine can be useful for balancing mood and managing anxiety (Landsberg et al., 2017). Pheromone therapy may also be useful in these cases (see below; Gunn-Moore and Cameron, 2004).

Conflict

Conflict is common in multi-cat households and can lead to stress. Conflict can be open with obvious signs (e.g. fighting) or silent where the signs are more difficult to recognize. Cats that feel threatened usually spend an increasing amount of time on their own, particularly when an assertive cat is present in the house, or may only interact with the owner when the assertive cat is elsewhere. Competition for resources (e.g. space, food, water, litter tray, safe places, attention) is a common cause of conflict and may start when a new cat is introduced or there have been other changes in the household. Having separate resources for each cat (preferably situated where they cannot be seen by other

Urinary crystal or urolith type	Nutritional adaptations
Struvite	■ A diet low in phosphorus and magnesium, with a reduced protein concentration (dogs only), and an acidic urine pH. The goal should be a urine pH of 6.4 in cats and 6.5 in dogs ■ In the long term, a urine pH of <6.2 is not recommended because in at-risk breeds (e.g. Miniature Schnauzer) acidic urine can precipitate calcium oxalate crystal formation (see Figure 20.1) Note: struvite uroliths are often associated with a urinary tract infection (UTI) in dogs. The UTI must be treated before dietary adaptations can be introduced for management of the uroliths
Calcium oxalate	■ A diet low in protein and sodium, and a neutral to mildly alkaline urine pH ■ Wet food types are advised ■ Increased water intake is required Note: calcium oxalate uroliths cannot be dissolved by nutritional adaptations but they can help decrease the risk of further formation
Cystine	■ A diet low in methionine (an amino acid of animal origin and precursor to cystine) (Osbourne *et al.*, 1999) and sodium, and a neutral to mildly alkaline urine pH ■ Wet food types are advised ■ Increased water intake is required
Urate	■ A low purine-producing diet, and a neutral to mildly alkaline urine pH ■ Ideal protein sources include vegetables, eggs and dairy. Diets containing proteins of animal origin should be avoided as they result in a greater concentration of purines in the urine Note: allopurinol is often prescribed in conjunction with the nutritional adaptations

Figure 20.3: Nutritional adaptations required to manage patients with various types of urinary crystals and uroliths.
(Data from Minnesota Urolith Center).

cat(s) in the household) can help reduce conflict. Cats should be provided with the opportunity to rest, hide, climb and scratch (both horizontally and vertically) without being disturbed. The use of elevated spaces such as shelves, boxes or beds may help to reduce conflict in multi-cat households.

Feeding

Some cats prefer to eat alone (i.e. if part of a multi-cat household), so it is useful to ensure that there is a quiet location where they can eat without being disturbed by other animals, people or sudden noises. Providing enrichment using puzzle feeders or hiding food around the house will allow cats to express predatorial behaviour and has been shown to be of benefit to some cats with FLUTD and related disorders (Dantas *et al.*, 2016).

Toys

Engaging in play activity, especially with owners, may decrease stress in cats. Encouraging cats to play with toys that are small and mimic prey characteristics can stimulate hunting behaviours (e.g. toy mice, feathered fishing poles).

Pheromone therapy

Pheromone therapy can be useful in many situations to help alleviate stress and anxiety in cats. Evidence shows that it can also be used to complement treatment for undesirable behaviours such as urine marking/spraying and aggression (Frank *et al.*, 2010; DePorter *et al.*, 2019). Products contain synthetic hormones that mimic the natural hormones that cats produce. They are available as electric diffusers that continually disperse pheromones into a given room and concentrated sprays that can be used for specific areas or objects (e.g. cat carriers). Diffusers seem to be more effective in some cases than the spray. One or more diffusers should be placed in the room(s) in which the cat appears to be most stressed, as well as near windows, doors, soiled furniture or litter trays. The use of pheromone therapy for cats with FLUTD is recommended during and after the implementation of MEMO.

Misconceptions for feeding a patient with lower urinary tract disease

Cranberries can help prevent disease

There is limited evidence to suggest that supplementing the diet with cranberries is effective in reducing the clinical signs associated with FLUTD (Colombino *et al.*, 2022).

Feeding a raw diet can help prevent disease

There is no evidence to suggest that removing grains and processed foods from the diet and instead feeding a raw diet can help prevent LUTD. Further, there are nutritional concerns associated with feeding some grain-free diets (see Chapter 4), home-prepared cooked diets (see Chapter 5), plant-based diets (see Chapter 7) and raw meat-based diets (see Chapter 6).

Preventing lower urinary tract disease

In many cases, there is little that can completely prevent LUTD from occurring. However, risk factors should be highlighted and the owner made aware of the clinical signs of disease so that swift action may be taken if they are identified. Correct nutritional adaptations and increased water intake, along with the treatment of any infections or underlying diseases, can help prevent further recurrences in many cases. In addition, feeding a urinary stress diet can reduce the short-term recurrence of FLUTD (Naarden and Corbee, 2020).

Communication with pet owners

LUTD frequently presents with clinical signs that owners find distressing, including pain, vocalization and the presence of blood in the urine. Owners should be reassured that swift veterinary attention and treatment can often resolve these clinical signs in a timely manner. In cases where the surgical removal of uroliths is required, the long-term benefits of dietary adaptations to help prevent recurrence should be explained.

Early detection in cats

Many cat owners do not observe their cat urinating and, therefore, early identification of clinical signs can be challenging. When LUTD is suspected, the use of special litter to help detect blood in the urine or changes in urine pH can be considered. These products contain granules that change colour when the urine is acidic or alkali and upon contact with blood, indicating that further investigation is required.

If a pet is straining to urinate without urine being produced, a urethral blockage may be present. This is an emergency and should be treated immediately.

Conclusion

Nutrition plays a key role in the management of LUTD cases. LUTD is common in both dogs and cats with some breeds predisposed to specific conditions. To make an appropriate nutritional recommendation, the type of LUTD present (including the composition of any uroliths) needs to be identified. An increase in water intake may be required in addition to dietary alterations and the administration of medications to help manage these conditions.

References and further reading

Bartges JW (2016) Feline calcium oxalate urolithiasis *Journal of Feline Medicine and Surgery* **18**, 712–722

Bartges JW and Corbee RJ (2023) Nutritional management of lower urinary tract disease. In: *Applied Veterinary Clinical Nutrition*, ed. AJ Fascetti *et al.*, pp. 412–440. John Wiley & Sons Inc., Philadelphia

Bartges JW, Osbourne CA, Lulich JP *et al.* (1999) Canine urate urolithiasis: etiopathogenesis, diagnosis, and management. *Veterinary Clinics of North America: Small Animal Practice* **29**, 161–191

Buffington CAT, Westropp JL, Chew DJ and Bolus RR (2006) Clinical evaluation of multimodal environmental modification (MEMO) in the management of cats with idiopathic cystitis. *Journal of Feline Medicine and Surgery* **8(4)**, 261–268

Chew DJ, DiBartola SP and Schenck P (2010) *Canine and Feline Nephrology and Urology*. Elsevier Health Sciences, Philadelphia

Colombino E, Cavana P, Martello E *et al.* (2022) A new diet supplement formulation containing cranberry extract for the treatment of feline idiopathic cystitis. *National Product Research* **36(11)**, 2884–2887

Dantas LM, Delgado MM, Johnson I and Buffington CT (2016) Food puzzles for cats: feeding for physical and emotional wellbeing. *Journal of Feline Medicine and Surgery* **18(9)**, 723–732

Defarges A, Evason M, Dunn M and Berent A (2020) Urolithiasis in small animals. In: *Clinical Small Animal Internal Medicine*, ed. DS Bruyette *et al.*, pp. 1123–1156. John Wiley & Sons Inc., Philadelphia

Defauw PAM, Van de Maele I, Duchateau L *et al.* (2011) Risk factors and clinical presentation of cats with feline idiopathic cystitis *Journal of Feline Medicine and Surgery* **13**, 967–975

DePorter TL, Bledsoe DL, Beck A and Ollivier E (2019) Evaluation of efficacy of an appeasing pheromone diffuser product vs placebo for management of feline aggression in multi-cat households: a pilot study *Journal of Feline Medicine and Surgery* **21(4)**, 293–305

Ellis SLH, Rodan I, Carney HC *et al.* (2013) AAFP and ISFM feline environmental needs guidelines. *Journal of Feline Medicine and Surgery* **15**, 219–230

Finke MD and Litzenberger BA (1992) Effect of food intake on urine pH in cats. *Journal of Small Animal Practice* **33**, 261–265

Forrester SD and Towell TL (2015) Feline idiopathic cystitis. *Veterinary Clinics of North America: Small Animal Practice* **45(4)**, 783–806

Frank D, Beauchamp G and Palestrini C (2010) Systematic review of the use of pheromones for treatment of undesirable behavior in cat and dogs. *Journal of the American Veterinary Medical Assocication* **236(12)**, 1308–1316

Güilersoy E, Maden M, Parlak TM and Sayin Z (2023) Diagnostic effectiveness of stress biomarkers in cats with feline interstitial and bacterial cystitis. *Veterinary Clinical Pathology* **52(1)**, 88–96

Gunn-Moore DA and Cameron ME (2004) A pilot study using synthetic feline facial pheromone for the management of feline idiopathic cystitis. *Journal of Feline Medicine and Surgery* **6**, 133–138

He C, Fan K, Hao Z, Tang N, Li G and Wang S (2022) Prevalence, risk factors, pathophysiology, potential biomarkers and management of feline idiopathic cystitis: an update review. *Frontiers in Veterinary Science* DOI: 10.3389/fvets.2022.900847

Landsberg G, Milgram B, Mougeot I, Kelly S and de Rivera C (2017) Therapeutic effects of an alpha-casozepine and L-tryptophan supplemented diet on fear and anxiety in the cat. *Journal of Feline Medicine and Surgery* **19(6)**, 594–602

Minnesota Urolith Center (2025) Treatment recommedations. Available from: https://urolithcenter.org/recommendations [Accessed on: 03/07/2025]

Naarden B and Corbee RJ (2020) The effect of a therapeutic urinary stress diet on the short-term recurrence of feline idiopathic cystitis. *Veterinary Medicine and Science* **6(1)**, 32–38

Nowak S (2022) Counselling clients on food bowl selection: what's the dish? *Today's Veterinary Nurse* **5(2)**, 18–22

Osbourne CA, Lulich JP, Kruger JM, Ulrich LK and Koehler LA (2009) Analysis of 451,891 canine uroliths, feline uroliths and feline urethral plugs from 1981 to 2007: perspectives from Minnesota Urolith Center. *Veterinary Clinics of North America: Small Animal Practice* **39(1)**, 183–197

Osbourne CA, Sanderson SL, Lulich JP *et al.* (1999) Canine cystine urolithiasis: cause, detection, treatment and prevention. *Veterinary Clinics of North America: Small Animal Practice* **29(1)**, 193–211

Pachel C and Neilson J (2010) Comparison of feline water consumption between still and flowing water sources: a pilor study. *Journal of Veterinary Behaviour* **5(3)**, 130–133

Schaible RH (1986) Genetic predisposition to purine uroliths in Dalmatian dogs. *Veterinary Clinics of North America: Small Animal Practice* **(16)1**, 127–131

Villiers E and Ristić J (2016) *BSAVA Manual of Canine and Feline Clinical Pathology, 3rd edn.* BSAVA Publications, Gloucester

Zanghi BM, Gerheart L, Gardner C (2018a) Effects of a nutrient-enriched water on water intake and indices of hydration in healthy domestic cats fed a dry kibble diet. *American Journal of Veterinary Research* **79(7)**, 733–744

Zanghi BM, Wils-Plotz E, DeGeer S, Gardner CL (2018b) Effects of a nutrient-enriched water with and without poultry flavoring on water intake, urine specific gravity, and urine output in healthy domestic cats fed a dry kibble diet. *American Journal of Veterinary Research* **79(11)**, 1150–1159

Online extras

This chapter includes:

● **A client information leaflet that is available to download and print from the BSAVA Library**

Access via QR code or: bsavalibrary.com/nutrition_20

Liver disease

There are two types of liver disease:

- Acute liver disease
- Chronic liver disease.

Liver disease can have many possible causes including infectious diseases (e.g. leptospirosis), non-infectious diseases (e.g. idiopathic chronic hepatitis), portal vascular abnormalities (e.g. portosystemic shunts), biliary tract diseases (e.g. bile duct obstruction), metabolic diseases (e.g. hepatic lipidosis), neoplastic diseases (benign or malignant tumours), vacuolar hepatopathies (e.g. due to corticosteroid therapy) and reactive changes secondary to other disorders. Liver disease results in the alteration and disruption of nutrient utilization, as well as loss of nutrient storage, causing nutrient deficiencies and malnutrition. Therefore, liver function must be supported via optimal nutrition throughout the course of the disease.

The effect of nutrition

With acute liver disease, the priority is to support the patient and allow time for the liver to regenerate and restore normal function. This is certainly achievable after a single insult that subsequently resolves. The liver has a large functional capacity and is capable of significant regeneration following damage. Hepatocytes retain the ability to proliferate, which means that functional mass can be restored even after >50% has been lost (Marks and Kathrani, 2023). In these cases, it is not usually necessary to feed a purpose-formulated dietetic food for liver disease. Optimal nutrition can be provided with a highly digestible, highly palatable, energy-dense diet, formulated to support recovery. With chronic liver disease, the dietary solutions depend on the clinical signs and cause of the condition. In these cases, the broad aims of nutritional management are to:

- Maintain and support liver function
- Encourage voluntary food consumption (anorexia is common in dogs and cats with liver disease)
- Maintain normal metabolic processes
- Correct electrolyte disturbances
- Support liver repair and regeneration
- Avoid toxic byproduct accumulation
- Avoid excessive production of ammonia
- Delay or prevent disease progression.

Essential elements

Energy

The diet should provide sufficient energy to meet at least resting energy requirements (RER) for patients with acute liver disease and maintenance energy requirements (MER) for patients with chronic liver disease (see Chapter 2).

Protein

Proteins are broken down to produce nitrogenous waste (i.e. ammonia), which is then converted by the liver cells into urea for excretion via the kidneys. In pets with liver disease, this process may be impaired, resulting in the accumulation of ammonia within the blood. Feeding dietetic foods containing proteins of high quality and high digestibility allows the nutritional requirements of the pet to be met from a smaller quantity of protein. This helps to reduce nitrogenous waste production. Plant-based protein sources (e.g. hydrolysed soya bean) produce less ammonia when catabolized than animal-based protein sources (Proot *et al.*, 2009), and foods formulated with such proteins are preferable.

Zinc

Zinc induces the copper-binding protein metallothionein, which decreases the amount of copper absorbed in the intestine thereby reducing hepatic accumulation (Fieten *et al.*, 2012). This may be particularly useful in cases of copper-associated hepatotoxicity (see below). To be effective oral zinc should be administered with food to minimize vomiting. For more information, see the *BSAVA Small Animal Formulary*.

Antioxidants

The inclusion of nutrients with antioxidant properties (e.g. glutathione) might be beneficial for combating the oxidative stress resulting from liver disease (Webb and Twedt, 2008). However, evidence for this is limited.

Suitable diet choices

The diet choice depends on the type of liver disease present and comorbidities of the patient. In very complex cases where multiple nutritional needs must be met, a suitable commercially manufactured product may not exist. In these cases, the best option would be to seek advice regarding dietary formulation from a person with an appropriate qualification (see Chapter 1).

Copper-associated hepatotoxicity

Copper-associated hepatotoxicity has been recognized in dogs, and less commonly in cats. This condition is associated with an inability to excrete copper or excessive dietary copper, leading to accumulation within the liver, chronic hepatitis and, eventually, cirrhosis. A genetic predisposition has been identified in some breeds, including the Bedlington Terrier (Thornburg, 2000) (Figure 21.1), West Highland White Terrier and Labrador Retriever. Genetic testing is available to screen for affected animals. Copper-associated hepatotoxicity may also be caused by non-hereditary mechanisms such as inflammation or fibrosis, although there is less evidence for this causing significant accumulation. Nutritional management includes the restriction of dietary copper and in some cases supplementation with zinc. However, not all studies have found a clear requirement for zinc (Fieten *et al.*, 2015).

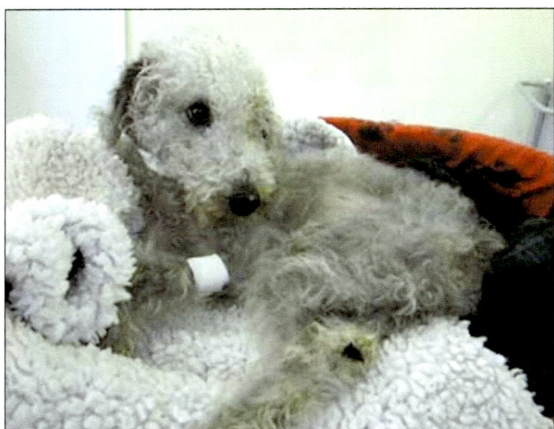

Figure 21.1: Bedlington Terrier with copper storage disease.
(Reproduced from the *BSAVA Manual of Canine and Feline Gastroenterology*)

Feline hepatic lipidosis

Feline hepatic lipidosis is a condition characterized by excessive lipid accumulation within the hepatocytes (Figure 21.2). It can result in hepatic dysfunction and cholestasis (Center, 2005). Cases typically present following a period of weight loss or anorexia. However, feline hepatic lipidosis may also occur in association with a systemic disease (e.g. pancreatitis), following a stressful event or be idiopathic. Nutritional management usually includes placement of a feeding tube, ideally an oesophagostomy or a naso-oesophageal tube in cases where the patient is unable to undergo general anaesthesia (see Chapter 13). Tube feeding is required to ensure delivery of sufficient energy to meet RER and the required concentrations of protein and essential amino acids. Intravenous fluid therapy with an amount of potassium tailored to the patient should also be provided.

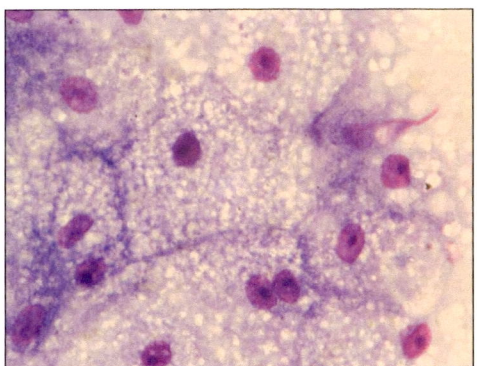

Figure 21.2: Cytological appearance of severe hepatic lipidosis in a cat. Note the great accumulation of fat globules in the hepatocytes. (Giemsa stain; original magnification X1000)
(Courtesy of Elizabeth Villiers)
(Reproduced from the *BSAVA Manual of Canine and Feline Gastroenterology*)

Portosystemic shunts and hepatic encephalopathy

Portosystemic shunts (PSS) are abnormal vascular communications between the portal and systemic venous systems, resulting in abnormal blood bypass of the liver. They can be congenital or acquired, the latter usually arising as a result of end-stage liver disease or hepatic fibrosis. A genetic predisposition to PSS has been identified in several dog breeds, including Yorkshire Terriers and Irish Wolfhounds (Van Steenbeck *et al.*, 2009). Clinical signs are usually due to hepatic encephalopathy (Figure 21.3). This syndrome results from bacterial breakdown of proteins to produce nitrogenous waste products (predominantly ammonia) within the intestinal lumen, which are subsequently absorbed, reaching the systemic circulation by passing through the PSS. Signs of hepatic encephalopathy may include: neurological signs such as disorientation, lethargy, ataxia and, in more severe cases, seizures or coma; gastrointestinal signs such as vomiting, diarrhoea and reduced appetite; increased thirst; and increased urination, resulting from derangement of neurotransmitter function in the central nervous system. Nutritional management involves feeding a diet with a low protein content. Diets using plant-based or dairy-based protein sources produce less nitrogenous waste products than diets with an animal-based protein source, and can decrease the clinical signs associated with PSS (Bauer, 1997; Proot *et al.*, 2009).

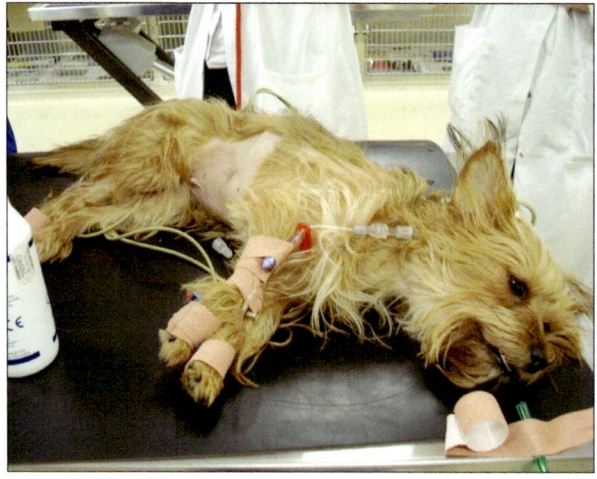

Figure 21.3: An 18-month-old female neutered crossbreed dog with severe hepatic encephalopathy due to a congenital portosystemic shunt.
(Reproduced from the *BSAVA Manual of Canine and Feline Gastroenterology*)

Misconceptions for feeding a patient with liver disease

Milk thistle is an important addition to the diet

Milk thistle contains silymarin (an antioxidant), which is suggested to be beneficial to those patients with liver disease. However, few studies have evaluated the efficacy of milk thistle in managing liver disease in dogs and cats, although reports have suggested positive effects on survival (Vogel *et al.*, 1984) and the protection of liver tissue against oxidative stress (Avizeh *et al.*, 2010; Hackett *et al.*, 2013).

S-adenosylmethionine is an important addition to the diet

S-adenosylmethionine (SAMe), a versatile molecule that plays a central role in methylation and glutathione synthesis within the liver, may be beneficial to those with disease. However, to date few studies have examined the benefits and further investigations are required (Anstee and Day, 2012).

Communication with pet owners

It is important that owners are provided with information about the specific condition affecting their pet and the nutritional adaptations that are required in order to help manage the disease. Details should also be given about the products and treatments that are recommended by the veterinary team and the supporting evidence for their use. Pet owners should be discouraged from searching the internet for treatments or supplements that have no scientific evidence of effectiveness.

Conclusion

Nutrition plays a key role in the management of liver disease cases. The liver is complex and performs a wide array of functions to help maintain health. Alongside medical treatment, appropriate nutritional management can help support liver function during periods of disease. The nutritional recommendation will depend on the type of liver disease present.

References and further reading

Allerton F (2023) BSAVA Small Animal Formulary, 11th edition – Part A: Canine and Feline. BSAVA Publications, Gloucester

Anstee QM and Day CP (2012) S-adenosylmethionine (SAMe) therapy in liver disease: a review of current evidence and clinical utility. *Journal of Hepatology* **57(5)** 1097–1109

Avizeh R, Najafzadeh H, Jalali MR and Shirali S (2010) Evaluation of prophylactic and therapeutic effects of silymarin and N-acetylcysteine in acetaminophen-induced hepatotoxicity in cats. *Journal of Veterinary Pharmacology and Therapeutics* **33**, 95–99

Bauer JE (1997) Diet selection and special considerations in the management of hepatic diseases. *Journal of the American Veterinary Medical Association* **210**, 625–629

Center SA (2005) Feline hepatic lipidosis. *Veterinary Clinics of North America: Small Animal Practice* **35**, 225–269

Fieten H, Biourge VC, Watson AL, Leegwater PAJ, van den Ingh TSGAM and Rothuizen (2015) Dietary management of Labrador Retrievers with subclinical hepatic copper accumulation. *Journal of Veterinary Internal Medicine* **29**, 822–827

Fieten H, Hooijer-Nouwens BD, Biourge VC et al. (2012) Association of dietary copper and zinc levels with hepatic copper and zinc concentration in Labrador Retrievers. *Journal of Veterinary Internal Medicine* **26(6)**, 1274–1280

Hackett ES, Twedt DC and Gustafson DL (2013) Milk thistle and its derivative compounds: a review of opportunities for treatment of liver disease. *Journal of Veterinary Internal Medicine* **27(1)**, 10–16

Hall EJ, Williams DA and Kathrani A (2019) BSAVA Manual of Canine and Feline Gastroenterology, 3rd edn. BSAVA Publications, Gloucester

Marchegiani A, Fruganti A, Gavazza A et al. (2020) Evidences on molecules most frequently included in canine and feline complementary feed to support liver function. *Veterinary Medicine International* **2020**, 1–7

Marks SL and Kathrani A (2023) Nutritional management of hepatobiliary diseases. In: *Applied Veterinary Clinical Nutrition*, ed. AJ Fascetti et al., pp. 319–344. Wiley Blackwell, Philadelphia

Proot S, Biourge V, Teske E and Rothuizen J (2009) Soy protein isolate versus meat-based low-protein diet for dogs with congenital portosystemic shunts. *Journal of Veterinary Internal Medicine* **23**, 794–800

Thornburg LP (2000) A perspective on copper and liver disease in the dog. *Journal of Veterinary Diagnostic Investigation* **12**, 101–110

van Steenbeek FG, Leegwater PAJ, Van Sluijs FJ, Heuven HCM and Rothuizen J (2009) Evidence of inheritance of intrahepatic portosystemic shunts in Irish Wolfhounds. *Journal of Veterinary Internal Medicine* **23**, 950–952

Vogel G, Tuchweber B, Trost W and Mengs U (1984) Protection by silibinin against *Amanita phalloides* intoxication in Beagles. *Toxicology Applied Pharmacology* **73**, 355–362

Webb C and Twedt D (2008) Oxidative stress and liver disease. *Veterinary Clinics of North America: Small Animal Practice* **38(1)**, 125–135

Online extras

This chapter includes:

- **A client information leaflet that is available to download and print from the BSAVA Library**

Access via QR code or: bsavalibrary.com/nutrition_21

Glossary

Term	Definition
Acid base	The body's balance between acidity and alkalinity
Acute disease	An illness that occurs suddenly and usually has a short duration
Adipokines	Cell-signalling molecules produced by the adipose tissue that play functional roles in energy/metabolic status
Adipose tissue hypoxia	Oxygen content of adipose tissue is decreased
Ad libitum (fed)	Food is available at all times enabling the pet to eat freely, whenever it chooses
Adverse reaction to food	This term is used for when dogs or cats develop clinical signs (usually related to the skin or intestine) as a result of something that they eat. It encompasses true food allergies (where the body mounts an abnormal immune response to a food component (usually protein)) and food intolerances (see below). This term is preferred because, in practice, it is very difficult to prove a true food allergy and, in fact, most are probably intolerances
Aerophagia	Excessive swallowing of air
Alternative protein-based diets	Commercially manufactured diets that use an alternative protein source
Altricial	Young are born helpless requiring significant parental care
Amino acids	Small molecules that are the building blocks of proteins
Analytical constituents	The nutritional analysis showing percentages of protein, fat, fibre and ash legally required on pet food packaging
Anorexia	Decreased or lack of food intake
Antiemetic	A drug that prevents or reduces nausea and vomiting
Antioxidants	Substances that protect cells against free radicals
Aspiration pneumonia	Occurs when food or liquid is inhaled into the airways or lungs causing inflammation and infection
Asymptomatic	Shows no signs of any problem
Beta cells	Cells within the pancreas that produce insulin

Term	Definition
Bioavailable	The amount of a particular nutrient that can be digested absorbed and utilized by the body after eating
Cachexia	Weakness and wasting of the body due to severe chronic illness
Carcinoma	A cancer that forms in epithelial tissue
Carnivore	An animal whose nutritional requirements are met by consuming animal tissues
Catabolism	The breakdown of complex molecules
Centile	A curve or line on a chart of measurements such as a growth chart. These are numbered according to the percentage of individuals whose measurements and gender fall below the line
Chronic disease	An illness that persists for a long time (e.g. at least 3 months)
Cobalamin	Vitamin B12 naturally found in foods. Has many functions including forming red blood cells and DNA
Colitis	Inflammation of the colon
Colostrum	The first milk produced after birth, which is rich in immunoglobulins (antibodies) and nutrients
Complex carbohydrates	A type of nutrient that is made up of sugar molecules strung together in long, complex chains. Usually found in foods such as peas, beans, whole grains and vegetables
Congenital	Disease or abnormality present from birth
Constipation	Painful or absent defecation caused by impaction of faeces in the colon
Cystitis	Inflammation of the bladder
Dam	Female parent of an animal
Deglutition	The act of swallowing
Demineralization	The process of removing minerals from hard tissues e.g. bone
Dietetic food	A diet that is formulated to support an animal with a particular disease or to prevent a disease from developing
Digestibility of food	How easily the body can break down the food into its constituents to be absorbed and utilized
Dilated cardiomyopathy (DCM)	A serious heart condition where the heart enlarges, its muscle becomes very weak, and the heart no longer pumps effectively
Dysrexia	A change in the pattern or behaviour of eating
Dystocia	Difficult or obstructed labour
Eicosapentaenoic acid	Omega-3 fatty acid that is required for various body systems including skin and coat, cognition and immune system

Term	Definition
Electrolytes	Minerals in blood and other body fluids that carry an electric charge
Endocrine	The complex network of glands and organs in the body that coordinate metabolism, energy level, reproduction, growth and development and response to injury, stress and mood
Enema	Medical procedure used to inject a substance, usually a liquid, into the colon; used to treat constipation
Enteropathy	A disease of the intestine, in particular, the small intestine
Exogenous	An external agent originating from outside an organism
Feline lower urinary tract disease (FLUTD)	A disease of the bladder and urethra of cats without an obvious underlying cause
Fermentable fibre	A type of fibre which is fermented in the colon into gases and active by-products by the bacteria in the gut
Fertility	The ability to produce young
Fluoroscopy	An imaging technique using x-rays to obtain real-time moving images
Folate	Vitamin B9; water-soluble and naturally found in many foods
Food intolerance	An abnormal response to a food component that is not caused by an allergy. Mechanisms of intolerance include the animal not having an enzyme needed to digest the component, the animal being particularly susceptible to a food component that others can handle, food spoilage (where the food goes off), or food poisoning (where the food is contaminated by a toxin or pathogen)
Free radicals	Highly reactive, oxygen-containing molecules that can damage cell membranes, enzymes and DNA. Considered to be a factor in the progression of disease and ageing; however, necessary for white blood cell function (oxidative burst)
Fundus (stomach)	The body or main largest part of the stomach
Gastric disturbance	Digestive disorders affecting the gastrointestinal tract
Gastric dilation volvulus (GDV)	Gross distention of the stomach with fluid and/or gas with gastric malpositioning
Gastroenteritis	Inflammation of the stomach and intestines
Gastrointestinal (GI) system	Composing the oral cavity, pharynx, oesophagus, stomach, small intestine, large intestine and anus
Genomic	Relating to the genes of a cell or organism
Gestation	The period that a female is carrying young *in utero*
Glucose	The main type of sugar in the blood which is the major source of energy for the body's cells

Term	Definition
Glucosuria	The presence of glucose in the urine
Glycaemic index	One of several values used to measure how rapidly the body digests or breaks down carbohydrates
Haematuria	The presence of blood in the urine
Haemorrhagic	Accompanied by loss of blood
Hepatic	Relating to the liver
Hepatic encephalopathy	A collection of clinical signs arising from the brain as a result of an underlying liver disease
Hepatic lipidosis	A disease in cats that arises due to the accumulation of lipid (fat molecules) in the liver
Hepatitis	Inflammation of the liver
Hepatopathy	A disease of the liver
Heterogenous	Composed of different constituents or dissimilar components
Hiatal hernia	An abnormal opening in the diaphragm that allows part of the stomach to bulge through into the chest
Hip dysplasia	Abnormal development of the hip joint
Homeostasis	The state of steady internal physical and chemical conditions maintained by living systems
Hormone	A regulatory substance produced in an organism and transported in tissue fluids to stimulate specific cells or tissues into action
Hydrolysed diets	Diets that have undergone hydrolysis. The process of hydrolysis breaks down proteins into small parts (polypeptides), making it more digestible and less likely to cause an adverse reaction. Often used to treat adverse reactions to food
Hyperadrenocorticism	A disease that occurs when the adrenal glands produce too much steroid hormone (cortisol)
Hypercalcaemia	An increased concentration of calcium in the blood
Hypercholesterolemia	An increased concentration of cholesterol in the blood
Hyperglycaemia	Increased blood glucose concentration
Hyperinsulinaemia	Increased blood insulin concentration
Hyperparathyroidism	Over-production of parathyroid hormone from the parathyroid gland
Hyperthyroidism	Over-production of thyroid hormone from the thyroid gland
Hypertrophic osteodystrophy	Developmental disease, autoinflammatory disease of the bones in young growing dogs
Hypertriglyceridemia	High concentration of triglycerides (fats) in the blood

Term	Definition
Hypocalcaemia	Low blood calcium concentration
Hypoglycaemia	Low blood sugar concentration
Hypoinsulinaemia	Low blood insulin concentration
Hypophosphataemia	Low blood phosphate concentration
Hyporexia	A decreased appetite
Hypothyroidism	Decreased production of thyroid hormone from the thyroid gland
Idiopathic	Refers to a disease with no identifiable cause
Immunity	The state of being protected against an infectious disease
Incontinence	Lack or voluntary control over toileting (urination or defaecation)
In utero	In the uterus
In vitro	A process that occurs somewhere outside a living body (usually referring to a test tube or culture dish in a laboratory)
Inorganic	Not consisting of or deriving from living matter
Intussusception	The inversion of one portion of the intestine within another
Ischaemia	Blood flow and oxygen is restricted to a part of the body
Ketoacidosis	An increased concentration of ketones in the blood causing it to become more acidic
Lactation	The process of making and secreting milk in the mammary glands
Laxative	A substance that loosens the faeces and promotes bowel movements (toileting)
Lethargy	General state of fatigue; lack of energy
Lipids	Broad group of organic compounds which include fats, waxes, sterols, fat-soluble vitamins, monoglycerides, diglycerides, phospholipids and others
Lymphangiectasia	Dilation, obstruction and/or dysfunction of the lymphatic vessels within the small intestine
Lymphatic system	A network of vessels in the body that drain a type of fluid called lymph from the tissues into the blood
Malnutrition	Lack of proper nutrition, usually occurring when the diet does not contain the right amount of one or more nutrients
Megacolon	Abnormal dilation of the colon
Melanin	A substance that produces pigment in skin, hair and eyes
Metabolic	Related to or deriving from metabolism within an organism
Metabolism	The chemical process of the body's ability to convert food and drink into energy

Term	Definition
Microbiome	Collection of all microbes such as bacteria, fungi, viruses and their genes that naturally live within the body
Mortality	Another word for death
Motility	The ability of small life forms to move independently, using metabolic energy
Neonate	A newborn infant
Neoplasia	Uncontrolled, abnormal growth of cells or tissues in the body
Nephron	Functional unit of the kidney consisting of a glomerulus and its associated tubule through which the glomerular filtrate passes before emerging as urine
Nitrogenous	Containing nitrogen in chemical combination
Non-fermentable fibre	Fibres not broken down by bacteria; adds bulk to faeces to make them easier to pass
Novel protein	A protein that is new to the pet (i.e. has not been consumed before)
Nutraceutical	A substance that is a food or part of a food supplement that is claimed to provide a health benefit
Nutritional assessment	A detailed, systematic evaluation of a pet's nutritional status and diet
Nutritional inadequacy	Intake of a nutrient or number of nutrients that is lower than the estimated average requirement
Obesity	A disease in which adipose tissue (body fat) has accumulated to the point that health is adversely affected
Oesophagus	The muscular tube through which food passes from the throat to the stomach
Omnivore	An animal whose nutritional requirements can be met either by consuming animal tissues or plants
Optimal	Ideal
Osmoregulation	The regulation of the osmotic pressure of bodily fluids
Osmotic diuresis	Increased urine production due to the presence of certain substances in the fluid filtered by the kidneys
Osteoarthritis	A degenerative joint disease
Osteochondrosis (OCD)	A disease of joints and bones that occurs during development
Oxidative stress	Imbalance of free radicals and antioxidant defences
Palatability	Refers to whether a food tastes good and is appealing to eat. Food that tastes good and is appealing to eat can be said to be highly palatable

Term	Definition
Pancreas	A glandular organ that produces digestive juices aiding in digestion, and hormones including insulin
Pancreatitis	Inflammation of the pancreas
Parenteral	Situated or occurring outside the intestine. When referring to administration of drugs, it usually means giving by injection
Parvovirus	A highly contagious virus mainly affecting dogs
Pathogen	A microorganism that has the potential to cause disease. Most pathogens are bacteria, viruses, fungi or parasites
Pathogenic	The potential for a microorganism to cause disease
Pheromone	A chemical substance created and emitted by organisms as odorants that may influence the behaviour or physiology of other members of their species
Plant-based diet	Comprised of cooked, plant-based ingredients
Polydipsia	Increased thirst
Polyphagia	Increased hunger
Polyuria	Increased urination
Portosystemic shunt	An abnormal connection (blood vessel of collection of blood vessels) between the portal system (vessels that connect the intestine and liver) and systemic system (the main blood circulation). This leads to blood from the intestine bypassing the liver
Postprandial	During or relating to the period just after eating
Prebiotic	A non-digestible food ingredient that stimulates growth/activity of bacteria in the colon, improving gut health
Probiotic	Live microorganisms providing health benefits by improving or restoring the gut microbiota
Proprietary food	Commercially manufactured food
Protein:creatinine ratio	A measure of the amount of protein in the urine which corrects for how dilute or concentrated the sample is
Protein-losing enteropathy (PLE)	A disease of the intestine accompanied by leakage of protein-rich fluid leading to its loss from the body
Pruritus	An itching of the skin
Purified diet	A diet that is formulated with a more refined and restricted set of ingredients
Purine	A chemical compound that is a building block of DNA and RNA
Pyloric stenosis	A narrowing of the opening between the stomach and small intestine
Pyometra	An infection of the uterus

Term	Definition
Refeeding syndrome	A shift in fluids and electrolytes that may occur in malnourished patients after starvation/fasting during a switch from catabolism to annabolism; potentially fatal
Regurgitation	The passive expulsion of matter from the mouth, pharynx or oesophagus
Remission	A period during which signs of disease are reduced (partial remission) or disappear (complete remission) with treatment
Restricted activity	A reduction in an animal's usual activities
Sarcoma	A cancer that begins in bone or soft tissues of the body
Sarcopenia	Progressive loss of muscle mass and strength; can occur with ageing
Satiety	The state or condition of fullness gratified to the point of satisfaction
Serotonin	A neurotransmitter with an integral physiological role in the human body; regulates various activities including behaviour, mood, memory and gastrointestinal homeostasis
Simple carbohydrate	A carbohydrate that contain one (monosaccharide) or two (disaccharide) sugar molecules
Sire	Male parent of an animal
Skeletal maturity	The age at which a cat or dog is deemed to be fully grown
Spondylosis	A condition causing degeneration of the intervertebral discs
Stoma	An artificial opening made into a hollow organ, and connecting it to the surface of the body. Examples include stomas in the trachea (windpipe), intestine or urethra (urinary system)
Stranguria	Straining to urinate
Supplementary	Additional information/medications that improve or enhance when given appropriately
Sustainability	The ability to maintain or support a process continually over time
Systemic	Affecting the body
Tenesmus	Straining. Usually associated with trying to pass faeces or urine
Thermoregulation	A homeostatic process that involves maintaining a steady body temperature
Torsion	The twisting of an object or organ (GDV)
Toxin	A naturally occurring organic poison produced by metabolic activities of living cells or organisms
Trachea	Also known as the 'windpipe'
Transit time (intestines)	The time taken for food to pass through the intestines

Term	Definition
Transition (of diets)	The time taken to change from one diet to another
Transverse colon	Part of the large intestine that runs across the body and connect the ascending and descending parts
Tyrosinase	Enzyme that controls melanin production
Uraemic syndrome	A collection of clinical signs that arise from the build up of waste products in the blood as a result of kidney failure
Uroliths	Bladder stones
Vomiting	Expulsion of contents from the stomach and small intestines
Weaning	The process of introducing solid food to young kittens and puppies
Zoonotic infection	An infection that can pass from animals to humans

Index